GUT FEELING

Why Diets, Exercise, and Shaming have Failed

Hamish Stuart

DARK
RIVER

To Andrea, Cara, and Aidan, for trying to keep me in line.

TABLE OF CONTENTS

INTRODUCTION

The thing is – the thing so many people don't get – is that no-one likes being fat.

It's not about a 'lifestyle choice'.

It's not about 'willpower'.

It's nowhere near as simple as 'eat less, exercise more'.

They say it is harder to be a vet than a doctor because animals can't tell you what's wrong with them. Well, fat people can talk but no-one listens to us.

No, really – they just talk *at* us. They think of ways to make money out of us. They ignore us because we don't do what they say. They would rather study the behaviour of rats than listen to fat people.

Yet current attempts at 'solving' the obesity crisis are just adding to the ever-escalating problems. It is time for fat people to have a voice, time for the obesity crisis to be addressed by 'doctors' rather than 'vets.' It is time for a new approach.

Billions of pounds and dollars are spent, millions of column inches written, months of TV and radio airtime broadcast, with people pounding out the same old messages and warnings about obesity. But, as the world faces up to a growing obesity crisis, there is one truth that is undeniable.

We have to change our thinking because diets are failing. A lot of thin people are putting pounds into their bank accounts, while a lot of others are putting pounds around their waists.

The first thing we need to address is obvious. There is a growing obesity crisis in the world, in the developed Western world in particular, and it affects all areas of society and age groups.

The second thing is equally obvious. What we are doing now is not working, and the people leading the efforts into fighting obesity are not succeeding. Their response to their failures is the blame game: blame the fat people for not doing as they say. That too, however, is making things worse.

Of course, there are thousands of books offering diets and explanations of the obesity crisis, thousands of classes and clinics running every evening, hundreds of academic studies, and thousands upon thousands of magazine, newspaper, and online articles extolling answers. TV programmes on the subject have grown rapidly, as have fitness DVD's and downloads; experts are breeding like rabbits. The bigger the 'crisis' gets, the more 'experts' there are – more and more people getting paid very well for failure. It feels as though anyone with a gimmick or a six-pack has a right to make money out of fat people.

Why are they failing? I think I know.

Almost all of the authors, writers, presenters, producers, experts, dieticians, and fitness trainers are thin. In their different ways, they are all basically telling fat people not to be so stupid – to be more like thin people, to be more like them. They are like a tourist, who does not speak a word of the local language, asking for something abroad – 'if the natives don't understand what you say in English, just say the same thing again . . . but louder.' If we keep getting fatter, then just shout at us louder. Instead, what the experts need to do is to try to learn our language.

But that would involve listening.

And believing!

And thinking!

So why is this book any different?

This is the book I wanted to read, as a fat person. I wanted us to have a voice, I wanted someone to explain what we are and why we are, but in terms we can understand. I wanted someone to offer realistic help. I wanted someone to stand up for us. I wanted thin people to read it so they could understand better. I wanted friends and family to read it so they would help constructively instead of nagging. I really, really wanted this book to be out there to help move the debate to a more realistic place, to start finding real solutions.

I do not want to be seen as someone making excuses for fat people. I am certainly not asking for any sympathy, but I do want understanding of why we are fat. I do want better help. I do want to shatter some of the widely held myths.

But who am I to write this book? A few things that I'm not, first of all. I'm not thin. I'm not a dietician, I'm not a nutritionist, I'm not a doctor or a medical research expert. I'm certainly not a fitness trainer. I'm not a psychiatrist or psychologist. I have not come up with a gimmick to sell. I have not made loads of money out of the diet industry nor am I likely to. I am not a celebrity, which worryingly also seems to be a qualification for pontificating on the subject these days. I don't have a catchy name for a faddy weight-loss programme. I'm not an Instagram model or social media 'star,' which again seems a worryingly common qualification. I have not lost enormous amounts of weight (either short term or long term) though I have lost some and more importantly kept much of it off.

I have worried, as I wrote this book, about who I am in comparison to all those scientists with their studies, their laboratories, and their rats. But then I look at the statistics to see the scale of their failures. I have come to understand myself better than they do - and the facts and figures back up the idea that I am far from unique. Hopefully, that means I understand *you* better than they do as well.

The joke goes that if you ask for directions in Ireland, then the local will begin by replying, "Well, I wouldn't start from here." The obesity debate, so far, has started from the wrong place. We concentrate on what makes thin people thin, but make little effort to find out what will succeed in making fat people less fat.

I can't say I've tried every single diet, but I've tried a lot of them alongside plenty of exercise regimes. Sometimes I have put on a little more weight and sometimes a little less, but the graph has always gone up – until recently when it has started going the other way a little thanks to some changes I will be able to stick with for the rest of my life.

There is a long way to go, there may just be an acceptable dead end, but either way, I hope I am on a better track. Anyone can do what I do and should do their version of it, but I'm the last person in the world to promise a miracle cure. There are no diets, no gimmicks, in this book.

So this is a journey, we have to get from A to B, from the current crisis to a better place. I have already explained we are starting from the wrong place and we are shouting loudly at the people with local knowledge, rather than learning their language.

We must start our journey by knocking down the main prejudices about obesity, key approaches which have failed for forty years and which actually stand in the way of making any progress.

On the route, we need to understand the real reasons why we are where we are. We need to understand our bodies and our brains.

Finally, we have to find answers to reach our destination – but answers that can work. That has to be a team effort. We need to address the global solutions for the global crisis, but we also need to look at ourselves.

We need to expose the myths, understand the reality and find a better future.

For this isn't some scientific theory to me; this is a daily reality. Quite simply, this is something about which I have a Gut Feeling.

PART 1: THE MYTHS

CHAPTER 1

Lifestyle Choice

"People who are overweight don't want unsolicited advice. Guess what. We know we're fat. We live in homes with mirrors."

Al Roker

We can all agree that the current approaches to obesity are failing, but so many people reading this will still be absolutely convinced that those basic "eat less, move more" messages are completely correct. They believe fat people are greedy, lazy and lack control. That's why we have to sort the myths from the reality before we can uncover what might be right. The myths become a barrier; at the expense of something else which might work better.

The first of these myths is that being overweight is a lifestyle choice.

This approach was perfectly summed up by a rather angry Sarah from Worthing speaking about serious obesity on a BBC radio phone-in. "This is not a disease, these people do not have a medical condition; it is quite simply biology. These people eat too much and exercise not enough. The cure for that, quite simply: eat less and exercise more."

It sounds so simple, so how can that message not have got through? In fact, worse than that, how can such a simple message appear to have backfired and made the problem worse?

British Government policy on obesity, as explained through the National Health Service website NHS Choices, would seem to broadly agree with Sarah – even if the phrasing is slightly more polite. "Obesity does not happen overnight. It develops gradually over time, as a result of poor diet and lifestyle choice."

You can find the same wording from Health Direct Australia. In turn, the US Department of Health and Human Services Surgeon General, David Satcher, MD Ph.D., phrased it like this in a 2001 Call to Action, "For the vast majority of individuals, overweight and obesity result from excess calorie consumption and/or inadequate physical activity."

Many people would put it more bluntly. One blog post from the Women's Health Research Institute at Northwestern University in Chicago stated, "Last weekend I noticed a billboard on the highway that read: 'Obesity is a disease, it is not a choice!' Nice way to avoid responsibility – put the blame elsewhere. Just remember, you can have a bowl of cereal in the morning, or a chocolate-covered donut. It's your choice... not some disease."

This reminded me of the movie The Book of Life, in which a fat boy gets stuck trying to fit through a small gap. His companion says he would have been fine without had had 12 doughnuts for breakfast. His defence was that he only had eight!

Sarah's anger was sparked by an earlier radio interview given by Professor Francisco Rubino, the chair of metabolic and bariatric surgery at King's College London, who told BBC Radio, "We have to change the public perception of obesity. The root of the problem is we completely misunderstand obesity; there is a lot of stigma against it. This is the last disease which is subject to prejudice and stigma.

"Many others have been in the past, in the centuries before… obesity is just the last."

Mental health, addiction, shell-shock, and dyslexia (amongst others) are just some of the areas over which we have gained, and are gaining, greater understanding and acceptance. We are discovering subtleties where there was once an assumed simplicity.

The approach to obesity which has failed for 40 years is to treat everyone the same. However, in reality, the more we understand the differences between us, the better we can treat the problem.

We have to stop treating those differences as excuses – an attempt to avoid deserved blame. We have to stop calling obesity a choice.

Are you convinced, like Sarah from Worthing and many others, that 'eat less, exercise more' is 100 percent of the answer? Certainly, all the evidence would show there must be more to it, or that simple message would have worked. Like all the best lies, the 'eat less, exercise more' message is based on a grain of truth – but it has still failed. We all need to understand that failure much better.

Force fed the wrong messages

When examining obesity, we need to strip-out the prejudicial language that influences the debate. There is a lot of pre-judgement in the way fat people are described, and it reinforces stereotypes and skewed thinking.

- Thin people eat, fat people shovel food into their gobs.
- Thin people act, fat people are lazy.
- Thin people think and take care, fat people are too busy stuffing their faces to consider the consequences.

These statements may resonate with you. You may well hold those views, or something broadly similar. You may be thin and blame fat people; you may be fat and blame yourself. But these statements help maintain the status quo. They reinforce attitudes, and it is attitudes – and ultimately derived actions – which need to change.

They say that if you keep doing the same thing, don't be surprised if you keep getting the same result. Whether you look at fat people with sympathy or distaste, with pity or blame, we can all agree we want a different result.

I am asking you to open your minds, listen to plenty of experts who have conducted years of research in their different areas, examine a new way of putting all that research together, and then think.

Over the years of failure to control my weight, I have listened to many of the 'experts'. I have tried to put what they say into practice, but I have failed. The reasons may be personal to me, but there is plenty of evidence that I am far from unique in my failures, and my feelings are the same as for many other fat people.

Blame is an easy thing. We are blamed for being fat, we are looked down on for being fat, we are denied medical treatment for being fat, and we are denied the chance to adopt children for being fat. That's just the start!

Being overweight affects fat people every second of every day, and part of that misery is how hard people work at not being fat, and not being able to enjoy the things they want.

Being obese is a bit like being an alcoholic – you never stop being one even if you have not had a drink for decades. Except being obese is harder than being an alcoholic – you can stop drinking completely, however tough that may be, but you cannot stop eating.

Each fat person faces their own battle, but there is more to this than individual choices. There are plenty of reasons why no-one would choose to be fat.

Global trends

There is a significant shift in the size of people across the world, and a recent study by Imperial College London[1] covering 186 countries, and just under 20 million participants, showed that obesity rates have risen in every country in the world over the last 40 years, without exception – including countries such as Somalia and Angola, where malnutrition remains an epidemic.

In a dictatorship such as North Korea, where there are many shortages for the common people, the increase is tiny. Japan is also low. Some other countries, with low increases, had high BMI rates at the start, places such as Bahrain and Nauru. In the Pacific islands of Micronesia and Polynesia, where size is not frowned upon socially in the same way as in the West, there have seen substantial increases with more than a third of men and more than half of women being classified as obese.

Globally, the average adult today is three times as likely to be obese compared to the average adult in 1975. The highest increase for men is in high-income, English-speaking countries; for women, it is central Latin America, though the rate of increase in high-income countries has slowed since obesity became a major issue around 2000.

To quote one conclusion of the study, "Present interventions and policies have not been able to stop the rise in BMI in most countries."

So, what's causing the rise? Fat people may be responsible for what goes into their mouths, but it seems clear there is more to it – factors outside the control of any individuals. Here are just a few examples often cited by scientists:

- The aggressive marketing of sugary drinks to all ages.
- Cheap convenience meals full of fat, sugar, and salt with low prices and questionable quality.
- Changes in farming and food production to make what we eat less nutritious.
- Growth hormones and antibiotics in the meat we eat.
- Changes in eating habits driven by multi-nationals, fast-food outlets, and supermarkets.
- Short-term diets.
- Government, education, and Health Service policies which – according to figures – are having no positive impact.

All these elements are part of the story. They all contribute to the amount and quality of what overweight people put in their mouths; they have all changed more in the last 40 years than the human body or mind.

The largest study held in the UK, backed by the Government with 250 contributing experts, concluded that excess weight was now the norm in what they called our 'obesogenic' society. They pointed to energy-dense and cheap foods, labour saving devices, the increased use of cars, and less active work. Dr. Susan Jebb of Oxford University, and the Medical Research Council, is one of the world's foremost experts and she believes we have to abandon the idea that obesity is down to individual indulgence.

"The stress has been on the individual choosing a healthier lifestyle, but that simply isn't enough," she said.

So if fat people are to be put on trial for obesity, it seems they should not be alone in the dock. The people driving those trends in society should be looked at as well: the politicians, the scientists, the farmers and – maybe more than anyone – the food industry.

Starting young

Being fat has a negative effect on every single part of your life. It affects your wealth, your health, your happiness, your relationships, your work, your success, your self-esteem, your hobbies, your entertainment, how others perceive you, friendships, your fertility, your parenting, your pain levels, incontinence… have I missed anything out? Quite a lot, as it happens, but that list will do for starters! And interestingly, many of the social implications of being overweight – the prejudices against fat people – run deep in society and start at a young age.

Research by Leeds University[2] in 2013 shows that children from the age of four are reluctant to have fat friends. In one particular experiment, researchers developed a specially made up picture storybook about a normal-weight character called Alfie. A group of four-year-olds read the book and, when asked, said they would be happy to make friends with Alfie. Indeed, when Alfie was redrawn as being in a wheelchair, the children maintained that they would be friends. However, when Alfie was drawn as fat, something dispiriting happened. Only 1 out of 43 Reception and Year 1 pupils said they would team up with Fat Alfie.

And the sex of Alfie made little difference. When Fat Alfie was changed to Fat Alfina, only 2 out of 30 pupils said they would team up with her. Professor Andrew Hill, who did the study, said: "This research confirms young children's awareness of the huge societal interest in body size.

"It shows that by school entry age, UK children have taken on board the negativity associated with fatness and report its penalties in terms of appearance, school activities, and socially.

"I think we have an underlying social commentary about weight and morals and that the morality of people is based on their shape.

"I think that is very powerful and kids are sensitive to it."

Hill believes the youngsters are picking up on a prejudice towards obesity that is all around them, from the opinions of their parents to TV shows which 'ridicule' the fat; such views almost certainly underpin weight-related bullying and victimisation.

Many parents of obese children say their youngsters are already socially isolated at the age of five.

Getting older

The downside of being overweight follows you into adulthood and affects your life chances. In fact, a World Obesity Federation report in 2018 declared stigma over obesity is the UK's most common form of discrimination.

Out of more than 1,000 obese adults who were asked about their experiences in the survey, 45% said they had felt judged when going to hospitals and the doctors. 32% had the same experience at the gym with 31% feeling judged at work. 62% said they thought those who were overweight were likely to face discrimination, compared to 60% due to their ethnic background, and 56% for their sexual orientation.

In 2013, research from a US-based executive education provider,[3] showed that fatter executives were perceived to be less capable, both in terms of job performance and their people skills. "Executives with larger waistlines and higher body-mass-index readings tend to be perceived as less effective in the workplace," the CLL study said

Santa Clara University business Professor, Barry Posner, told The Wall Street Journal he could not think of a single overweight Fortune 500 chief executive. "We have stereotypes about fat. So when we see a senior executive who is overweight, our initial reaction isn't positive," he added.

Typically, the lesson drawn from the survey was that overweight managers needed to hit the gym, not that others needed to re-assess their negative assumptions about overweight managers.

Fat people punch below their weight in the workplace. There are many studies into weight discrimination at work based around the National Survey of Midlife Development in the United States. In 2005, researchers found that around a quarter of obese workers and a third of very obese workers reported discrimination that they put down to their weight and appearance.[4]

Two years later it was reported overweight people were 12 times more likely to report discrimination than thin people, obese people were 37 times more likely, and severely obese people 100 times more likely.[5] Several studies of legal cases of wrongful sacking show that weight, rather than performance, was the deciding factor in overweight people losing their jobs.

'They would say that, wouldn't they' might be the response of some, but that's missing the point. If being overweight is supposedly a lifestyle choice, would anyone really *choose* to put themselves in a position where they feel 100 times more likely to be discriminated against?

Further research offers more insights.

Several studies show that obesity has a negative impact on wages. For example, John Cawley of the University of Wisconsin[6] found in 2004 that being an extra 64 pounds (four-and-a-half stone) above average weight correlated with 9% lower wages. That 9% was the equivalent of 18 months of more education, or three years more work experience. Another survey showed the difference in wages for the severely obese to be almost 20% lower for white men, and 24% for white women.[7] (It is a more complicated picture for people from ethnic backgrounds because more factors are involved, though the trends are the same.) It is a similar story in studies across the European Union; women, once again, are affected slightly more than men.[8]

To test perceived prejudices against fat people – that they are less conscientious, less agreeable, less emotionally stable, and less extroverted – Michigan-based researchers[9] conducted studies in 2008 to examine whether such assumptions were accurate. They found no significant differences in those personality traits between fat people and thin people. Other factors such as age and gender played a bigger role.

Rebecca Puhl of the Rudd Center of Food Policy and Obesity at Yale University has covered the stigma of being fat in great detail, pulling together several reports across different areas.[10] As she makes clear, "These findings help challenge commonly-held stereotypes about negative personality traits of overweight employees." Namely, that fat people are lazier, less productive, and more likely to be off work sick.

Whilst there are some successful self-made large ladies and gentlemen that spring to mind, the more weight you carry, the harder it is to climb up a large company's greasy pole. Corpulence is not conducive to corporate success.

And, of course, there are industries where fatness is truly frowned upon! Entertainment is one, and it was all rather brilliantly summed up by the late Star Wars actress Carrie Fisher, who returned to her Princess Leia character 38 years (and a few more pounds) after first starring in the role. She was told to lose about two-and-a-half stone before filming started.

"They don't want to hire all of me – only about three-quarters," she told Good Housekeeping magazine.

"Nothing changes, it's an appearance-driven thing. I'm in a business where the only thing that matters is weight and appearance.

"That is so messed up. They might as well say get younger, because that's how easy it is.

"We treat beauty like an accomplishment, and that is insane.

"Everyone in LA says, 'Oh you look good', and you listen for them to say you've lost weight. It's never 'How are you?' or 'You seem happy!'"

Brilliant.

The burden of weight

If you watch the many TV programmes about fat people, interviewees are often moved to tears when discussing their weight and the impact on their lives. The only other subjects that bring as many tears to the TV screen usually involve death or fear.

I was struck by the comments of one lady interviewed on the American TV programme The Weight of the Nation. She was in her twenties and pretty large. She admitted she had never had a sexual relationship. "I do not want a chubby-chaser, I want someone who wants me for who I am. I suppose food is my boyfriend."

She cried.

How often have you heard the comment, "So and so would be really good-looking if he/she was not so fat." Or, "He/she has a really attractive face under all that fat."

It is a particular problem for women in the world of dating. The nasty side is a trend called Pull a Pig, where men date plus size women for a bet or because they think it 'funny.' Researchers have shown that overweight women are less likely to be chosen through a dating site than those with a history of drug problems![11] Yet, there are also plenty of studies which show that obese and non-obese people are equal in terms of the quality of their relationships.

There is a bit of a common thread developing here – the difference between perceptions of fat people and reality.

Put simply, prejudice trumps truth. Or as Hartung and Renner put it in Frontiers in Psychology in 2013, "Today overweight and obese individuals face discrimination in almost every domain of living."

That's quite some 'lifestyle choice'.

Salad days

If I had a pound for every time a thin person in the world has quietly said to a friend or family member in a concerned voice, "You have to *decide* you want to change – that would help you lose weight," then I would have more money than Bill Gates. My other favourite is, "Why don't you eat more salads – they are terribly filling, you know!"

Funnily enough, I understand why they say it. If you are a thin person who puts on a couple of pounds every now and then, you probably like salads, find them relatively filling, and it is no great hardship to eat one occasionally instead of fattier food. It works for you and, as a result, you cannot get your head around why fat people do not do something so simple.

I went out for lunch once with a couple who decided to order a single salad between them to share, because it was too big and filling for one person! My jaw hit the floor so hard I struggled to chew my chips.

Part of the misunderstanding is the idea that fat people eat for pleasure; we enjoy something naughty but nice and cannot control ourselves. We are prepared to sell our bodies for the pleasures of overeating, a bizarre self-sacrifice on the altar of fatty food.

If you are basically thin, then you *do* eat some nice things purely for pleasure. The pleasure can even be additional to the taste; it's something you enjoy because you have earned it, you deserve it, you can get away with it. A little bit of what you fancy can make some people self-affirmingly smug. If you found yourself putting on weight, you could easily give up those little extras for a while, so you can't understand why anyone would be different.

That's not how I eat. It's not *why* I eat.

I do not eat for pleasure; I get guilt. I'm not that bothered about the taste. Given the choice between something pleasurable and something filling, I would choose the latter every time. Pleasure would not even enter into the decision-making process a tiny, little bit. I could get pleasure from a biscuit or a slice of cake – but I can only get satisfaction from a packet of biscuits or a whole cake.

I get much more driven to overeat functional foods, things that help me avoid feeling bad. I have no problem eating 'healthily' but even eating 'healthily' is not good for you if you eat too much of it. For instance, I have no strong feelings in terms of short-term pleasure between the taste of cherry tomatoes and shortbread, but I know the latter will be more satisfying.

I compare it to the Roman Catholic concept of Purgatory, where – after you die – your un-saintly soul has to go through a period of purification before you can be considered for a place in heaven. So, Purgatory is where your soul is condemned to roam the earth powerlessly while waiting to go to heaven – or hell. That is what being hungry feels like, an aimless unhappiness that dominates your life until you can get to somewhere better – in other words, somewhere to eat.

I have a feeling at the back of the throat. It's as though that's the only part of my body which matters, like an itch you can't scratch; it's hard to think or concentrate on anything else. Then there is an emptiness in the stomach before the frontal lobes of the brain feel as though they are going into overdrive.

It is a desperation, an uncontrollable urge. I wish it was not there. I wish it did not take over my life until something happens to satisfy it.

When I eat, I know what I am about to do is wrong for me and unhelpful. Apart from anything else, being fat hurts your joints, makes life uncomfortable, and means you cannot do everything you want. No-one would make pain a lifestyle choice. But on another level, it is the only thing that allows life to return to normal. A content mental state is the result of giving in to food urges; continual restlessness is the result of refusing. It is possible to choose the latter for short periods – minutes, days, weeks, months, possibly even a small number of years – but the first option gets harder and harder to ignore. It gets ever more difficult to cope with being continually restless.

If you do not get those feelings, or only a pale shadow of them, then of course you think fat people are being stupid and greedy. They would be both those things if they had the same level of urges as you. Instead, we need to recognise there are key differences – and there is plenty of science to back that up.

Unfortunately, a taste of food only seems to trigger an even stronger desire. Eating is then really, really hard to stop. There is an obvious hormonal explanation that once the Pandora's Box of desire hormones have been released, they cannot be put back again easily. For example, I have a problem with leaving food; I have to eat it all even if that food is someone else's salad.

It's not always someone else's salad.

No 'one size fits all' solution

The above is personal to me, but once again the explanation is backed up by the science. Finnish researchers at the University of Turku[12] have studied "how eating stimulates the brain's endogenous opioid system to signal pleasure and satiety." Roughly translated that means eating gives you a buzz in the same section of the brain as heroin, while also making you happy and feeling full.

That's interesting and encouraging, but not half as interesting as the next bit. They discovered that the brain releases endorphins (pleasure hormones) when you eat a pizza. No surprise there. However, they went on to discover that the brain releases even more endorphins when you have a tasteless nutritional drink.

"The magnitude of the opioid release was independent of the pleasure associated with eating," reported Eurekalert.

A tasteless nutrition drink lights up the pleasure centre of the brain more than pizza. In other words, obesity absolutely is not about doughnuts for breakfast. It is about providing enough nutrition to satisfy the brain, not about pleasure chasing.

The report goes on, "The opioid system regulates eating and appetite, and we have previously found that its dysfunctions are a hallmark of morbid obesity. The present results suggest that overeating may continuously overstimulate the opioid system, thus directly contributing to the development of obesity. These findings open new opportunities for treating overeating and the development of obesity."

Confirmation that there is so much more to obesity than a lifestyle choice. There is something treatable, once we accept treatment is necessary. So, if we can forget some of the stigmas around obesity, maybe even treat it as the last misunderstood disease, we can move forward in a more effective way. We also need to analyse exactly what we are dealing with.

There are many different reasons for being fat; there are different categories of fat people, and, perhaps appropriately, there is no 'one size fits all' solution. But there are a few basic principles that will help us start to recognise where solutions can be found.

It is like positive and negative discipline; appropriately, we need more carrot than stick. If you tell someone to try something they cannot do, they rebel, they go the other way. It is easier to admit to a bad attitude than failure or weakness. Feeling a failure, feeling powerless, is actually another stimulant to do the things that make you fat. It stops fat people looking for the things they *can* do – it reinforces hopelessness. Fat people have a lot of self-defence mechanisms, and eating is often one of them.

You cannot band everyone who is not at optimal weight together. In fact, trying to treat all fat people the same is a substantial part of the problem – solutions for one group are not solutions for another. This is a hugely important point because so much weight loss advice is based on 'This is what worked for me.'

Of course, in scientific terms, there is a wide range of numbers available on the Body Mass Index (BMI) which is just a combination of height and weight, but I would band people together in more social terms – even fat people are not just numbers!

My first category is **Thinnies**. These are people who find it easy to remain relatively thin; in fact, they would find it genuinely hard to put on any serious extra weight. Unfortunately, they dominate the high profile and high-level positions in society, so the very people with the lowest level of understanding have a disproportionately loud voice in the debate.

The second category is for people who are just a few pounds overweight, or even a couple of stone, often for an obvious reason. These people are not naturally fat so a small change will bring big results. I call these the **Lifestyle Fatties.** The concept of Lifestyle Choice may not be the right way of putting it, but Lifestyle Change would certainly be effective for them.

The third category are not only physically fat, they are large framed and also mentally attuned to being large. They are forever trying to do the right thing, but somehow keep getting it wrong. They will put on a little bit of weight each year (anecdotally an inch a year around the waist), but it might be an inch every two to five years. In the case of some women, this may have followed childbirth as the trigger for weight gain. It is a huge daily concern to them, but they cannot stop themselves. This is the group who are most demonised in society. I'll call these the **Proper Fatties,** which is a lot politer than a lot of the names they face.

Of course, the first two groups have more of a 'choice,' or rather – I would argue – weaker urges.

However, much of the book will deal with the problems facing this final group because they are the most under-represented. They are perceived as the biggest problem, but their case is the hardest to address – partly because solutions that work with the first two groups are also applied to them despite continual failure. If we can do it the other way around, and meet their problems head-on, then the solutions will be even easier for the other groups.

I would also put myself in that final group, grossly obese, obscenely fat, to borrow some of the comments that fly around. These are the people who have not been given a voice, who have been most written-off. We want to find an answer.

Thin people believe we lead some gloriously hedonistic life, stuffing our faces out of selfish greed, gorging on chocolate donuts for breakfast. It's not like that in reality, but to explain this argument properly and appropriately we need to put more flesh on the bones.

Let's start by addressing the issue of willpower…

CHAPTER 2

Willpower

"None of us wanted to be the bass player. In our minds, he was the fat guy who always played at the back."
Paul McCartney

I think thin people are lucky. No more, no less – although they think they have better judgement and stronger willpower. That is part of the problem, why so much of the advice is wrong. In a curious way, the worse the obesity crisis gets, the more thin people feel smug and superior.

The whole Willpower Myth – that we can solve the obesity crisis if fat people showed more mental strength – is really about letting thin people pat themselves on the back. If fat people are mentally weak then, by definition, thin people are mentally strong; and that's a nice thought.

Hopefully, you may now accept that being overweight is not a deliberate choice. It is driven by bodily feelings which a thin person does not get to the same degree as a fat person. However, many will still respond by arguing we just need to show more willpower (like them). The brackets are usually left unsaid.

A University of Chicago survey in 2016,[13] described by lead researcher Jennifer Benz as, to her knowledge, the most comprehensive view of Americans' beliefs about obesity, showed that three-quarters of the wide range of people questioned, both thin and overweight, thought the main cause of obesity was a lack of willpower.

The New York Times reported the findings like this, "Researchers say obesity, which affects one-third of Americans, is caused by interactions between the environment and genetics and has little to do with sloth or gluttony. There are hundreds of genes that can predispose to obesity in an environment where food is cheap, and portions are abundant.

"Yet three-quarters of survey participants said obesity resulted from a lack of willpower. The best treatment, they said, is to take responsibility for yourself, go on a diet and exercise.

"Obesity specialists said the survey painted an alarming picture. They said the findings went against evidence about the science behind the disease, and showed that outdated notions about obesity persisted, to the detriment of those affected."

The survey questioned 1,500 people of all sizes; 94% of those who took part in the survey had tried to lose weight through diet or exercise. A quarter had tried many diets, and one-in-seven (around 15%) had tried more than 20 diets.

As Dr. Louis Aronne, the director of the Comprehensive Weight Control Center at Weill Cornell Medicine and New York-Presbyterian, explained, "Trying 20 times and not succeeding — is that lack of willpower, or a problem that can't be treated with willpower?"

No excuse

The aim of knocking down the arguments about willpower and elevating other elements, such as environment and genetics, is not to give fat people an excuse for being weak-willed. The point is that if we accept environmental and genetic contributions to obesity, we can also try to find environmental and genetic *answers* to reducing obesity.

If we look in the right areas, we are more likely to find the right answers.

As Dr. Stuart Flint, a psychologist with a focus on the psycho-social effects of obesity, told Sky News: pointing the finger is easy, gaining a full explanation is harder.

"We know there are over 100 different factors that contribute to overweight and obesity and it's time the public were really given the information they deserve... that obesity is complex... it's not simple," he said.

The belief in 'willpower' is a barrier we need to get over. For a start, willpower is a vague and much-misunderstood concept. It is about a person's ability to control his or her actions consciously. We like to think willpower is a positive; we like to boast about it, we think it represents an example of our mental strength. We like to think we have lots of it; it is a sign of good character.

So it may come as a surprise to many that psychologists can influence and predict our behaviour to prove we have very little willpower, estimated at just 5-10% of our actions. Even worse news, when we really do show willpower, it often has a negative effect. To put it more simply, genuine willpower is small and makes us do things worse!

A research university in Ohio[14] showed that when we actively resist nice food, our performance levels drop because we fail to concentrate as effectively on the tasks in hand.

They set problem-solving tests for people sitting at a table with a bowl of radishes on one side and a bowl of chocolate, cookies, and sweets on the other. One group was told they could eat the radishes, but not the chocolate, cookies, and sweets; another group could eat as they wished – (I'm not sure they needed to enforce a 'no radishes' policy.) There was also a control group with no food on the table.

The problem-solving test involved drawing a figure in a continuous line without crossing the line or re-tracing. Unknown to the participants, it was designed to be impossible. They were not being measured on their ability, but to see how hard they tried and how they coped with failure. The group restricted to the radishes (they could not eat the nice food) did much worse in their reactions than those who could eat the nice food and those with no food at all, both in terms of how hard they tried and in controlling frustration. To paraphrase slightly, when the going got tough, those eating the cookies and sweets got going. The radish group were distracted by the nice food they could not eat, and had to utilise their willpower to stay on task. The conclusion was that consciously avoiding 'bad' food through willpower negatively impacts performance.

Yale University's John Bargh has undertaken decades of research on how easily our actions can be influenced by external factors. Along with Tanya Chartrand, then both at New York University, they wrote, "…most of a person's everyday life is determined not by their conscious intentions and deliberate choices but by mental processes that are put into motion by features of the environment and that operate outside of conscious awareness and guidance."[15]

They talk both about the daily manipulation of opinions and actions. For example, people rub their face more when with someone else is rubbing their face. People using the same mannerisms tend to like each other more, which is knowledge that people often deliberately exploit when dating or selling. They also looked at the refusal of people to believe their own actions are anything other than fully self-controlled.

The classic example taught on most management courses is getting someone to stay in a room after a fire alarm goes off, just by putting them in with a group of actors and actresses who are briefed to be nonchalant and not move. It is classic herd effect and amazing how often we can be influenced to react in a way that is illogical.

Because self-control can play such a big part in distracting us from efficiently carrying out any other task, humans have needed to minimise the impact of willpower in order to aid survival. Psychologist Roy Baumeister, of Florida State University, along with Kristin Sommer, concluded in 1997 that we only successfully use conscious self-control for around 5% of the time.

Cognitive therapist Dawn Walton, the author of The Caveman Rules of Survival, told the Huffington Post, "Most of us believe we have conscious control of our choices. It's simply not true. Your subconscious is in charge for at least 90 percent of the day.

"That part of your brain is primitive, emotional, and quite frankly, stupid; but it means well. It is always looking to make you feel better. So when you find that eating that bar of chocolate makes you feel happy, even for a moment, you know that comes from your subconscious."

Baumeister and Sommer argue that most people estimate their own self-control at 90+%, a complete reverse of all the research evidence. We continually talk about making choices, though we are far more pre-programmed than we imagine.

Other researchers offer similar perspectives.

Dr. Susan Jebb of Oxford University told The Independent that the obesity crisis cannot be pinned to a "national collapse in willpower. ... It's something about our environment that has changed," she said. "You need, in some cases, a superhuman effort to reduce your food intake. Is that their fault? I don't think it is."

Professor Michael Cowley of Monash University, Australia, told The Daily Mail, "People may have a tendency towards obesity even before they eat their first meal. Obese people are not necessarily lacking willpower. Their brains do not know how full or how much fat they have stored, so the brain does not tell the body to stop refuelling. Subsequently, their body's ability to lose weight is significantly reduced."

Obesity expert Dr. Donna Ryan, Professor Emeritus at the Pennington Biomedical Research Center in Baton Rouge, Louisiana, said, "It's frustrating to see doctors and the general public stigmatize patients with obesity and blame these patients, ascribing attributes of laziness or lack of willpower to them. We would never treat patients with alcoholism or any chronic disease this way. It's so revealing of a real lack of education and knowledge."

Fat people themselves often give in to the perception that we lack the right attitude. One person, in a Fat Class I went to, ranked his determination to lose weight as just five out of ten, something that was leapt on by our instructor as an area that could be positively improved. The fat person's logic was that as he was fat, so he cannot have attached much importance to trying to get thin. He would rather admit to bad decision-making than mental weakness. Increase the importance and decrease the weight, seemed the simple equation.

However, the same person was prepared to work a night shift, then jump straight in his car, drive a couple of hundred miles, risk traffic gridlock because of 'once-in-a-lifetime' road closures, sleep in his car outside the meeting hall rather than going home and risking the traffic jams a second time, all to make the next meeting of our Fat Class. Does that really sound like five out of ten commitment to you?

When 'willpower' came easy

From a personal perspective, I have had long periods when 'willpower' has been really tough but also had periods when 'willpower' – in terms of eating – has come easy. There were two particular periods of a few months, after knee operations, when my appetite plummeted. I only wanted portion sizes less than half my normal size. It was great! Of course, I lost weight, but also I could eat what I liked – lots of 'naughty but nice' foods because I only wanted small quantities. I craved well-balanced food, including lots of vegetables. I could eat what I wanted, as much as I wanted, when I wanted, and still lose weight; all because my body had more urgent things to worry about. It was glorious.

It was so much nicer than my normal existence; my normal desires. If I had a choice to live like that all the time, then I would, in a flash. It was far, far more pleasurable than any food binge I have ever had.

Unfortunately, my body's hormonal levels (something we shall explore later in the book) resumed once the physical recovery was completed. The first time my lack-of-appetite happened, I thought (for a while) it could be the new me; I was naive enough to think it might be something I could control, it could be a permanent change with a little willpower – but of course it didn't work like that.

I also find 'willpower' comes extremely easily in other areas, such as gambling, drugs, or smoking. Or, to put it more accurately, I have no urges to do any of them – which makes them pretty easy to resist. Because I have no interest in gambling, I could lecture gamblers and tell them not to be so silly. I would put forward lots of good reasons, but the bottom line is my advice would be ignored because I have no real understanding of what drives gamblers. There are plenty of parallels in the obesity debate – lots of diet advice comes from people who know as much about putting on weight as I do about gambling.

One smug newspaper columnist boasted about there being "willpower, and then there is my willpower," before banging on about their superiority in relation to food and drink. Of course, they had it the wrong way round. Their urge is a tiny, invisible itch whereas mine is a nasty, big, red, swollen, poisonous bite. Theirs can be easily ignored or sorted with a quick scratch, mine will irritate the hell out of me, or worse, unless there is an effective antidote or cream. Or cream cake.

So to sum up, the vast majority of fat people are not happy being fat. We hate it, it is horrible. We also understand the consequences.

People show extraordinary willpower to lose weight, sometimes to lose weight again and again and again. And yet the end result is almost always failure – just how depressing do you think *that* is? Pretending not to care – to be happy fat people – is sometimes easier than confronting that reality of continual, heart-breaking failure.

I'll answer Dr. Aronne's question from the start of this chapter ("Trying 20 times and not succeeding — is that lack of willpower, or a problem that can't be treated with willpower?"). It's *not* lack of willpower, it *is* a problem which cannot be treated with willpower.

Despite that, there is only one treatment for obesity which is generally accepted – to go on a diet. So, next, I need to show why diets are not only failing as a treatment, they are making things worse.

CHAPTER 3

Diets

"If we are not meant to have midnight snacks, why is there a light in the fridge?"

Facebook Meme

The world's biggest report on diets, by scientists from UCLA in 2007[16] concluded that going on a diet was one of the best predictors of future weight gain. You haven't read that wrong, going on a diet reliably indicates that you will probably weigh *more* in the long run.

So, quite simply, I believe every person pushing a short-term diet should be charged with fraud. Some may be well-meaning, they may be pushing something they sincerely believe in, but the overall figures show what they are doing is fraudulent.

Let's face it – all the evidence shows that for most people, going on a diet is like going to a loan shark. You get what you want in the short-term easily enough, but you repay that with added interest over the long-term.

That may seem a strong statement, but the facts are overwhelming.

How can I possibly say that I am right when there are hundreds of thousands of experts around the world – many highly qualified, many medical doctors, some who have been doing decades of research in this area – who think something completely different?

Simple… because people are getting fat in increasing numbers and yet (if you remember the US survey of a representative cross-section of 1,500 people mentioned in the last chapter) the vast majority (94%) have already been on a diet. In other words, high numbers of people are trying a vast range of diets, and they are not working in the long-term. If no-one wants to be fat, and we had a successful way of preventing it, then no-one would be fat.

So, despite the multi-billion pound industry, the thousands of medical research teams, the massive amounts of magazine and news coverage, the huge number of books and apparent easy fixes, we have not found a solution. The only pounds lost by the population as a whole have come out of peoples' wallets. Research, classes, theories, books, articles, medical advice – they are all going up, and so is the average weight.

The perfect diet does not work

The last thing the diet industry needs is something that works. If that happened, the industry would die out overnight. The perfect commercial diet works short-term to get people to invest their money in following that advice, but if it worked long-term, then it would be self-defeating.

The other thing which is exposed by the vast amount of money spent on diets and diet advice is that fat people are desperate to lose weight. Desperate. The number of gimmicks we chase, the number of classes we take, the amount of time, effort, and money we spend all prove that.

We will try things which may damage our health, which will be deeply, deeply unpleasant, which will dramatically affect our bodily functions in potentially bad and uncomfortable ways. We really will try almost everything and, of course, the less it works, the more we try. We try poisons; we even take things that could kill us in horrible ways – just to try and find a way we CAN lose weight.

Selling the idea that there could be an easy fix may be commercially successful – that we can be like the thin, good-looking people pushing a fantasy – but rarely is it successful in the real world. In fact, it is damaging; it puts fat people off doing the right thing in order to pursue all these gimmicky wrong things. It sends out confused messages and puts the wrong type of pressure on people. That pressure can lead to unhappiness, depression, and even death.

The long and short of it

The figures show that most people who lose weight in a diet will end up heavier a few years later. The shorter the time period of the survey, then the lower the numbers who will have regained the weight (the figures suggest 30-50% of people will have regained their weight in two years).

But longer-term studies, over a two-to-five year period, consistently show a higher return of weight in the years after a diet; for studies that look at people over four years or more, more than 80% of people will have packed the pounds back on.

Bear in mind, as well, that many of those studies include people with average BMI indexes (below 30) and many of younger ages including students. Furthermore, many studies rely on the self-reporting of weight even though all the evidence shows people regularly underestimate it – either accidentally or deliberately.

Some studies are commissioned by the diet industry themselves, though even those supposedly 'positive' studies show an incredibly low success rate – for instance only 16% of the most committed, self-selecting sample of Lifetime Members of Weight Watchers remained at their target weight after five years, according to a 2007 report published in the British Journal of Nutrition by long-term Weight Watchers consultant Dr. Michael R Lowe, of Drexel University, Philadelphia.[17]

These were people who started with an average BMI of 27.5, so had very little to lose in the first place. Only half stayed at 5% less than their original weight after five years, again a staggeringly low return given that these were the best of the best, who started with so little to lose. Even Lowe admits these are a "fraction" of the overall Weight Watchers membership.

When you take factors such as timescales and under-reporting into account, I would argue that the real failure rate of diets for *Proper Fatties* over a period of years is mighty close to 100% – but there is more bad news.

If you suddenly lose weight then the body panics; it thinks it is not getting the food it needs and sets about becoming ultra-efficient at storing extra fat. It goes into what is called *Starvation Mode*. Eventually, it just means that a dieter's body stores more calories from the same meal compared to a non-dieter – calculated as the equivalent of 20% more calories for the dieter – even though the two meals are identical.

It sounds mad, but the bottom line is that dieting makes your body around 20% less efficient at losing weight. Fat people on a diet are already eating a fraction of what they could eat, or would like to eat; now they need to reduce that figure by a further 20% – 500 calories a day for a man and 400 calories a day for a woman – just to counteract the negative impact of going on a diet in the first place.

There are different estimates for this figure of metabolic change, but my personal experience confirms it is certainly progressively harder to lose weight, even when you carry on doing the same things.

The figures are explained by a person's changing metabolic rate, which is largely based on size, which drops as your weight drops, as does the percentage of muscle mass within that size. More muscle means more energy used and a higher metabolic rate. Many rapid weight loss diets inevitably involve losing muscle.

The Biggest Loser

There is a pin-up poster of the 'Eat less, Exercise More' Diet Brigade.

The Biggest Loser (nice positive name) is a TV programme around the world which takes various fat people, applies traditional diet and exercise approaches, and follows their short-term weight loss. The dieters talk about their new determination/willpower, get fed a couple of lettuce leaves a day, and are then flogged in exercise – or something like that.

It is a vehicle for smug dieticians, fitness trainers, and programme-makers to show how clever they are in 'helping' these poor fat people lose weight. It underlines all the damaging myths and prejudices in a very high-profile way. It always irritated me, even before the report (below) came out.

Before we get to the report, though, if taken at face value then the Biggest Loser approach appears to work; at least over the short-term of the TV programme. Everyone loses weight to a reasonable degree. To take one example in America, Season 8 winner (they really did more than eight seasons of this?) Danny Cahill lost 239 pounds, more than 17 stone or 100 kilograms. By any measure that is remarkable! It made great TV as this thin man burst through, literally, a paper image of his former self.

Pats on the back all round at the end-of-the-series party of fruit and vegetable smoothies.

Now, the bit they don't show on the programme.

Scientists led by Kevin Hall, from the National Institutes of Health (NIH), Maryland, USA, published a follow-up study tracking the Season 8 contestants six years later. 13 out of the 14 regained weight in that period, four weighed more than before the programme, and the 'winner' – Cahill – had regained 100 pounds.

For 10 out of the 14, the numbers pointed to improvement up to a point, but there were more worrying elements of the study. Because the body's metabolism essentially rebels against the weight loss, the metabolism slows down during and after the diet period. Taking Cahill as an example, six years later, his metabolism uses 800 fewer calories per day than would be expected for his size. He has to reduce his daily calorie intake by around an extra third just to keep his weight steady.

Hall and his team advocated the theory of the body having its own 'set weight' and the metabolism adjusting to that set level. While that removes the blame aspect of obesity, it is also a concerning theory that offers little hope for the future. The bottom line is the study emphasises that it is incredibly difficult for fat people to lose weight. But then we knew that as well . . . if anyone had listened.

Plainly that 'set weight' has changed in the last generation; the average BMI index has gone up a couple of points, so once again that is either the case of several million people independently changing or some wider trends taking effect.

It all shows that diets make our bodies *more* efficient at storing fat. Yo-yo weight loss and gain are *less* healthy than consistency, and diets are a part of the problem – they appear to make us fatter and less healthy.

Quantity, not quality

Then there is the fact that the majority of commercial diets are just about losing weight, rather than the type of weight you lose. Weigh yourself every day, or at least every week – that is the bedrock of all diets. Take pictures of yourself to put on the fridge for motivation. Do a chart to show your weight loss. That is the sort of advice flying around, even before you start going to the weekly self-flagellation of a slimming class.

However, simply losing weight is not the issue; it is the type of weight you lose that counts.

You do not want just to lose fluid, as some quick-fix diets do. You do not want to lose muscle weight, as the majority of diets do, as that stores up health problems. Muscles also help use up calories and increase your metabolism, so a 'bikini/six pack plan diet' that involves short-term weight loss, including muscles, will be counter-productive in the long-term. You just want to lose body fat, but that needs to be measured separately. Almost none of us have the resources to check on that every week.

The British Dietetic Association has an annual top five celebrity diets to avoid at all costs; diets plugged by various Hollywood stars, pop stars, models, etc. They include no-sugar, only eating Kale cabbage and chewing gum, a special 400 calorie coffee (instead of eating), food supplements and pills. I would recommend looking it up for a laugh and a lesson.

Speaking about these and other fad diets, Sian Porter, consultant dietitian and Spokesperson for the BDA, said:

"We hear it all when it comes to the latest way to shed pounds from the good to the bad, to the down-right dangerous! When people need medical advice, they go to their GP and when people have a toothache, they go to their dentist, but some people will believe almost anything and anyone when it comes to nutrition, food and diet.

"The bottom line is, if it sounds too good to be true, then it probably is. If you have to pay out for a DVD or book or product that will unlock the secrets of losing weight, this can be a good indicator that the only pounds you will be losing will be out of your wallet. The simple fact is, there is no 'wonder diet' just as there are no 'super foods' and no one diet fits all. What is super, is the way many marketing machines coin certain phrases to make you think there is some magic wand approach to losing weight."

There is perhaps a parallel with diets and the world of golf. Golf equipment is substantially better today than it was previously, and makes the game easier than it has ever been. There is more advice flying around from the world's top players, all the superstar coaches, and better and cheaper ways of passing on that advice through the internet; but the average handicap of the club player has not gone down, and in some parts of the world it has actually gone up.

The world's best players have used the equipment to get much better, to the point they can destroy many traditional courses, but that has not trickled down to club amateur level. If the equipment and the advice are so much better than ever, that seems strange. But if you think about the number of regular one-to-one lessons with coaches and how people practice the same amount as before (maybe even less in our busy age) – then it makes sense.

Do you need to walk the walk?

The fact there is so much bad diet advice on offer begs the question – do you need to have done something yourself to be able to talk about it? In most walks of life, the answer is typically 'yes'. To be a sports pundit, you will have likely played at the highest level, to have been through the heat of the cauldron to be respected for your understanding of the sport.

There are plenty of sports players who resent the comments passed on them by journalists who have never played at the highest level themselves. There is a feeling that there are certain judgments (critical ones usually) that journalists should not make because of that lack of knowledge. It is like Chelsea and former England footballer John Terry rather ridiculously saying he would only accept criticism from former players who were as good as (or better than) him. Curiously, no-one has ever questioned my right as a sports journalist to flatter, but that is a different point.

The principles apply in almost every other walk of life; to talk about politics, you need to have been a politician, political academic, or seasoned observer; to talk about a crisis on the other side of the world, you need to have been there or seen an equivalent crisis somewhere else. To talk about fashion, you have to be fashionable yourself.

So the principle that it helps to have been there, done it, and got the T-shirt, is pretty well established.

Except in the area of obesity. In this area, the 'experts' are people who have not been there, not done it, and not got the 4XL T-shirt.

The vast majority of the experts pushing diets are thin and, generally, they have always been thin. They may have lost a few pounds, possibly a stone or two, but these are Lifestyle Fatties. They can talk about how they avoid getting fat, but they have no real knowledge of how Proper Fatties get fat. These people confuse their knowledge of getting down from 13 stone to 11, with what it is like to be 20 plus stone. They have lots of answers, but they are answering the wrong questions. They may have put on weight, but none of them have the underlying body shape close to mine or many other fat people. None of them have our hormone balance.

The only people who truly understand the issue are fat people, but they are not trusted to be part of the answer. In the United States, an obesity forum was set up to help inform the President and Congress; one of their meetings was shown on Weight of the Nation. It was a room of people who were experts on the theory, but not the practice.

Short, sharp shock

A short, sharp diet will typically only work for people who are relatively thin, because their overall rate of weight gain is so slow that the occasional burst the other way buys them enough time. You might decide that if you can keep your weight down by going on one easy diet each year, then surely anyone can. However, if the aim is to reverse long-term weight gain then short, sharp diets are as effective as a chocolate teapot (rather appropriately).

The problem is when you are in the 'inch a year' brigade of the expanding waistlines, or some group that sees a similarly steady rise in weight. Then, the short, sharp diet brings in the risk of the 20% more efficient storage of body fat.

There are plenty of studies that show diets do not work, but the biggest ever done was the 2007 UCLA report mentioned at the start of the chapter. In the paper, in American Psychologist, researchers went through 31 diet studies with a fine-toothed comb to come up with some pretty comprehensive findings.

Traci Mann, a UCLA Associate Professor of Psychology, and the lead author of the report said, "You can initially lose 5 to 10 per cent of your weight on any number of diets, but then the weight comes back. We found that the majority of people regained all the weight, plus more. Sustained weight loss was found only in a small minority of participants, while complete weight regain was found in the majority. Diets do not lead to sustained weight loss or health benefits for the majority of people.

"What happens to people on diets in the long run? Would they have been better off not to go on a diet at all?

"We concluded most of them would have been much better off not going on the diet at all. Their weight would be pretty much the same and their bodies would not suffer the wear and tear from losing weight and gaining it all back."

The report quoted one study that found both men and women who took part in formal weight loss programmes ended up putting on more weight over a two-year period than those who had *not* taken part in a weight loss programme.

In turn, one of the longer-term studies showed 83% of those measured for more than two years put on more weight than they had lost, while one found that 50% of dieters weighed more than 11lbs above their starting weight five years after the diet.

Furthermore, the adverse health benefits of losing and gaining weight – including heart disease, stroke, diabetes, and altered immune function – provides additional consequences.

The background to the UCLA research was the question in America about whether health insurance should cover dieting as a treatment for obesity. Medicare had deleted the words "Obesity is not considered an illness" in 2004, which opened the door to funding treatment if it could be considered an illness. The conclusion was firmly that diets would not be an effective treatment worth funding, thus trying to close the door again.

One final quote from Traci Mann (my favourite, actually) revealed this opinion. "My mother has been on diets and says what we are saying is obvious." In other words, all these studies by thin people were just proving what overweight people already know.

A million calories a year

Dieting has created an obsession with daily calorific intakes. But if we take a moment to look at things over a wider timescale, some interesting observations emerge.

Let's assume the average man needs a million calories (realistically over a million once you build in normal activity), around three-quarters of a million for the average woman, and just over half a million for a child.

I find the larger figures help put things in perspective. For instance, one whole giant bar of chocolate would be an irrelevance over a year, about

0.1%, so a one-off binge at the end of a bad day would not have any long-term impact. However, a habit, say half a small bar of chocolate each day, would be about 20% of your total recommended annual intake and clearly have a massive impact.

The obesity crisis has led to people questioning Christmas Day, with people ringing up phone-ins suggesting that anyone fat would be irresponsible to eat a full Christmas dinner. Even if someone manages to eat 7,000 calories on Christmas Day – Turkey is a low-fat meat and the meal includes loads of vegetables – that would still represent just 0.7% of their annual intake over the 365 days. There are far bigger problems than 7,000 calories on Christmas Day. A Mars Bar every day may help you "work, rest, and play", according to the advert that ran years ago, but it would be 102,200 calories over the year. I find the longer-term view helps identify habits rather than one-offs.

Sugary drinks are seen as a major cause behind the increase in obesity, particularly in America where the consumption levels of full-fat soda drinks are higher. According to the Harvard School of Public Health, the percentage of sugary drinks imbibed as part of the US daily calorie intake has more than doubled to 9%. For children between the ages of 6 and 11, in the US, the calorific percentage has increased by more than half again. Sugary drinks are the top calorie source for teenagers, narrowly edging out pizzas.

Rightly, these are scary figures.

A 330ml can of Coca-Cola is 139 calories, including the infamous ten spoonful's of sugar, but the Coca-Cola website suggests various ways of burning off that energy including 11 minutes of vigorous salsa dancing, half an hour of yoga or Pilates, or half an hour of walking. They have a calculator to show you how long you need to do a wide variety of sports to burn off those 139 calories. It even works out that you need zero minutes of that long list of exercises to compensate for the calories in a Diet Coke – though that drink has other issues.

A small can of Red Bull is 110 calories, and most fizzy or energy drinks are in the three-figure number of calories category.

You can 'buy' extra calories through exercise to the extent that Olympic rowers, for example, need 6,000-8,000 calories a day to stop their bodies eating muscle to get the extra energy their training regimes require. I did an interview with an international sportsman, once, as he finished his cheesecake, kindly rushing the interview between the end of lunch and the team bus departing. These people need a carefully-monitored amount of sugar and calories or their athletic performances suffer. They are still supremely fit, and their body/fat ratios are ridiculously low.

They would even be allowed Christmas dinner every day without the killjoys getting involved, but athletic nutrition is far more advanced than offering any one meal. Because they need plenty of calories, the emphasis of sports nutrition is on the quality of the food. I was told one anecdote by someone who spent time eating the same food as a group of elite sportsmen and who lost weight over that period without trying. They could eat as much as they liked, but it was all good quality, well-balanced food.

Mind you, there was another international sportsman who went through a period of having his meals provided for him in cardboard boxes as a way of keeping his focus, nutrition, and weight on the straight and narrow. They included plenty of such delicacies such as beansprouts – although he complained that the cardboard box was the best-tasting bit!

Work in progress

How do you define if a diet works? All too often, success is seen as getting people to start – generally at some cost – rather than worrying about the end result. Fat people can always be blamed for failure, rather than the dietitian.

Diets rarely address long-term issues. Almost all of them have a time span, with an end in sight. If they marketed themselves as a long old slog for the rest of your life, then they would be much less successful. Of course, there are recommendations to take the lessons on board at the end, but the main selling point of diets is their ease. No-one has made millions on the back of a diet that will be deeply unpleasant to follow, for an ongoing period of misery; I missed that marketing campaign if there was one.

Eat as much as you like and still lose weight – now that really is a money-spinner. And that is the claim of many diet pills. There is one diet pill that claims amazing results, as long as you also stick to 1,500 calories a day and plenty of exercise at the same time. I was going to say you would have to be stupid not to see the pointless expense of adding the pill but, in fact, a better word to use would be desperate. Most fat people are desperate enough to try almost anything. Raspberry ketone, fat-burning pills, acai berries – if they really worked, they would sweep the world, but of course they don't.

They can even be dangerous cons – some of the so-called fat burning pills, such as DNP, speed up the metabolism so badly that people are basically boiled alive from the inside. One victim was found dead in an ice bath; the result is truly horrible. Think how bad someone's body image depression must be to take that poisonous risk. Has that person really made a 'lifestyle choice' to be fat if they kill themselves trying to be thinner?

One of the latest gimmicky diets is the 3-Day Diet or Military Diet, or even the 3-Day Military Diet – whatever you call it when it is barking mad. The selling point of this diet is ice cream, not just because I screamed in anger when I first heard of it.

The diet is meant to help people lose up to 10lbs in three days, and I am sure it is successful in terms of losing weight. I'll give it the most credit I can possibly contemplate and say it might be a useful tool for people who are not really fat, who are planning for an imminent important day.

Might.

However, for anyone who is fat, it is lunacy. Such a short-term bounce has no long-term permanence. So what are the attractions? Well, you can eat ice cream, did I mention that? Ice cream on a diet, who'd have thought it – guaranteed column inches with that one! Then it is only three days; surely anyone can put up with a bit of hardship for three days – even fat people! And there is substantial weight loss, up to 10lbs, more than half a stone in such a short space of time. What's not to like?

And you can eat ice cream, did I mention that bit?

Here is the most calorific of the three days.

Breakfast | 1/2 Grapefruit, 1 Slice Toast, 2 Tablespoons of Peanut Butter, and Coffee or Tea Total: 297 calories, 39g of carbs, 10g of protein
Lunch | 1/2 Cup of Tuna, 1 Slice of Toast, and Coffee or Tea Total: 174 calories, 14g carbs, 23g of protein
Dinner | 2 Slices of any type meat, roughly 3 ounces, 1 Cup of Green Beans, 1/2 Banana, 1 Small Apple, and 1 Cup of Ice Cream Total: 598 calories, 76g carbs, 34g of protein
Daily total: 1069 calories, 129g of carbs, 67g of protein.

The calorie intake reduces over the following two days – obviously trying to lull the body into a false sense of security with that bumper intake on day one! The overall intake over the three days is less than 3,000 calories – but you do get to eat ice cream every day.

Of course, you should lose weight in that period – because the overall calorific intake is low – but one of the many issues with it is the idea that simply losing weight is the objective. How much of that weight loss is fluid? How much is muscle as the body converts it to find the energy it needs? In both cases, that will be weight gained as soon as things return to normal.

Perhaps, more importantly, that diet will create cravings in fat people. In the unlikely circumstance that I was able to stick to that diet for three days, the cravings for food that would build up for day four would be incredible. The only parts of that daily diet that would go any distance towards filling me up would be the two slices of toast, tuna (if I liked tuna), three ounces of chicken, and a small cup of green beans.

So the weight I would lose would be mainly water and muscle, and I would create cravings that would likely mean replacing all those calories within 24 hours, 48 hours at the outside, of the diet's end. In turn, I would contribute to reducing my body's efficiency by 20% making any weight loss far harder in the future.

The Atkins conundrum

The Atkins Diet is one of the most successful weight-loss regimes in dieting history. At one stage, it was estimated that one-in-eleven North Americans were on it. The diet plan effectively meant cutting out carbohydrates, one source of energy. The diet was much more complicated than that, including chicken, tomatoes, vegetables, and so on, but people I knew just took it to mean a regular fry-up. Now a fry-up with three sausages, four rashers of bacon, two eggs, baked beans, and two hash browns would be thoroughly satisfying for most people, too much for many, but all that would come to 1298 calories (approximately). In other words, two of those a day would keep you around the recommended daily limit, and a small amount of exercise or activity would mean you would lose weight in theory. Of course, if you were already dieting and therefore your body is 20% less efficient, then you could have one-and-a-half of these fry-ups to last the whole day.

However, the key to success was the controversial claim by Dr. Robert Atkins that this particular method of burning fat without carbohydrates used up more calories in its own right; he estimated it added almost 1,000 calories to the daily allowance because of the "metabolic advantage". The theory was that low insulin levels meant the glucose was burnt off faster.

Many people found it worked for them, but the Atkins Diet succeeded commercially for two main reasons. One, it was pleasant to go through (certainly compared to other diets); and two, it satisfied the brains of fat people and actually worked in terms of losing weight. It went out of fashion once a different analysis of the long-term health effects of fat intake was publicised. In the end, the medical journal The Lancet got involved[18] and stated there was no such metabolic advantage. The Lancet report offered the opinion that it worked because the food was so monotonous that, after a while, people would simply cut down the quantities they ate.

Dr. Robert Atkins died in 2003, following a head injury falling on ice, and since 2010 – a New Atkins Diet has emerged. It represents a more balanced approach that still relies on a diet with few carbohydrates. It looks nowhere near as enjoyable to go through, or easy to stay on, though. Of course, it is nowhere near as successful, commercially, as the halcyon 'fun' diet days.

Funnily, the basic premise of the Atkins diet is making a comeback with rather better research to back it up. Harvard's David Ludwig, in his book Always Hungry? is one of a growing group of proponents of a high-fat, low-carbohydrate diet, which involves similar principles, albeit in a slightly different balance to the Atkins Diet. Ludwig also argues, backed up by research studies, that such a diet does have a modest metabolic advantage in the low hundreds of calories. Crucially, it depends on the right type of fat.

However, there is also 2018 research on mice in Zurich, Switzerland, to consider.[19] It suggests that such a high-fat, low carbohydrate diet may increase insulin resistance and so lead to Type 2 diabetes.

Leaving the scientific disagreements aside, for now, suffice it to say that, in commercial terms, the Atkins Diet illustrates the Holy Grail of diets. It had quick results, was easy for fat people to do, and had a scientific gimmick. If you can persuade fat people it really is their metabolism that is the problem, and hang out the promise of an extra 1,000 calories a day without doing any damage, then you have the commercial blockbuster it became for a while. When its popularity collapsed, the Atkins Nutritional company went bust, before re-emerging in a smaller form. Sadly for them, espousing a more balanced diet makes things less commercially successful.

Bad diet = good business

There are plenty who can show how a bad diet equals good business! The simple truth is that all short-term diets have a problem.

You see, anyone can come up with a diet which will lose weight in the short-term. Simply count up the calories of various foods until you come up with a figure somewhere between 1,000 and 1,500 and tell people to eat that each day. You can do the calculations to include some treats, one small chunk of chocolate a week, for example, to make it more attractive. You can even offer ice cream once a day...

So, these days, what separates the successful from the unsuccessful is not the diet itself, but often the attractiveness of the person pushing that diet. Men with six packs; women with slim, svelte bodies, all good-looking facially; the message is that by following their Wellness,

NutriBullets, spiralizer, Body Coach, clean living methods – at great expense – you too can look like them. In this social media world, the attractiveness of the person pushing the diet is more important than the long-term reality of what they are pushing.

Unfortunately, you cannot find a way around the hormonal imbalance of fat people that easily. To illustrate this, I will give a personal example. I went on the Cabbage Soup diet for a while. It involved making a massive pan of cabbage soup and eating some of it whenever hungry, whilst sticking to small, low-calorie meals the rest of the time. I quite liked the soup and, while it did nothing for my rear emissions, the diet worked in terms of weight.

At a conscious level, I was happy; eating that way was not a problem. It reduced guilt, and it was working. However, it did not work in terms of satisfying the brain at a subconscious level. The cravings for other foods got stronger and stronger as my brain felt it was being denied all sorts of things it wanted in terms of quantity and quality. I was having virtually none of the food that gave me a satisfied feeling, replacing it with cabbage soup.

Eventually, the food-control part of my brain went slightly doolally.

I compared the cravings to those of a pregnant woman, which was laughed at by my wife and other women, but I honestly cannot imagine any craving being stronger. The craving took over my brain; it took over all thought processes. The back of my mouth was permanently salivating as though preparing for food. The need for food became my only cognitive process, especially when out and about in the car or – even worse – when going shopping.

One day, I went into a supermarket and bought a bag of five jam doughnuts and a packet of Jammie Dodgers biscuits. I went back to the car, drove to a quiet corner of the car park, and scoffed the lot. After that, my brain could return to normal life.

This became a semi-regular occurrence as I stayed on the diet. I could think of little else before these occasional binges and afterwards became the only time my brain was able to relax and concentrate on other things. I imagine it was a bit like a drug addict getting a fix (there are substantial similarities in terms of the chemical reactions in the brain). I knew it was a wrong and stupid thing to do; I knew it would undo the good that was happening in terms of weight loss. At least, I could save money by choosing the jam doughnuts that were close to their sell-by date – there was no danger of them going stale by the time I reached my car and even less danger of them lasting any longer than that!

However, that is not the real point of this story.

The funny thing is that after coming off the Cabbage Soup diet almost two decades ago, I have not had a single jam doughnut. Not one. I have plenty of vices in food terms, but funnily enough jam doughnuts are not one of them – apart from that month to six weeks when I could not leave the supermarket car park without having finished all five in a family pack.

Now, even if I am going to eat something really bad for me, like a cheesecake, or biscuits or apple crumble, even when I walk past the doughnuts section and see they are reduced for a quick sale, I never have doughnuts. Never. It isn't some willpower thing; I just don't fancy them anymore. And it's not because I had so many that I've gone off them. If I was offered one, then I would eat it happily enough; but that 'desperation' went the second the last drop of cabbage soup went down the sink.

It is interesting that doughnuts offer pretty much the perfect balance of sugar and fat that the cabbage soup diet was denying my body. Take away that need, and you take away the cravings.

Incidentally, it is worth pointing out that the cravings of a pregnant woman may be a source of humour, but they generally make perfect sense from a nutritional point of view. If a mother-to-be wants broccoli and ice cream, or chocolate with marmite, then those foods are strong in the vitamins, protein, sugars, and fats that her body needs for the pregnancy. The demands may defy logic on a rational level, but they make perfect sense in terms of body balance and the health of the child.

All in the mind

The above just goes to show the power of the brain's cravings – and how diets can actually have a negative effect by upsetting the balance of the brain. Diet 'experts' count calories, they don't calculate hormones, and that is why they fail time after time.

Most fat people have been on a wide range of diets; they will have tried almost everything at some point or another. I am no exception; it is a statement of the obvious that none of them have worked and I will not go through them in great detail because they all missed the mark, and none of them work for the majority in the long-term.

There are so many different diets, so many different approaches. British mind specialist and hypnotist Paul McKenna did a series about Thinking Yourself Thin, accompanied by a book that was no doubt pretty successful commercially. I watched the programme with some excitement, thinking there might be a chance of seeing my mental issues addressed. Maybe hypnotism could alter the chemical balance of my brain, for example?

One of McKenna's first pieces of advice was to put your knife and fork back down on the table between mouthfuls. The theory was that if you ate more slowly, then you would feel full after eating a smaller portion. I have heard similar theories, including that you should throw away all your big plates and only use small plates to encourage smaller portion sizes. Or that you should take small mouthfuls and chew for longer.

There is a similar school of thought that suggests you wait before eating; you 'respect' the food and by thinking about what you are about to eat, you end up being satisfied by less. You have the weird sight of people staring at the food they are about to eat for a couple of minutes. That's fine if it's too hot, madness if you are letting it go cold, and barmy if you think that will really affect the brain's acceptance or otherwise of what you are eating.

Problematically, the idea that you can think or reason yourself into eating less misses one main point. Eating is driven from the gut and the brain, not the eyes. Chemicals are released to the brain from the stomach and intestines on the basis of satisfaction gained, not the speed of eating, and not because the plate looked full, or there was a wait before getting stuck in. Eating is not a rational thought process; it is a primeval urge. We are not programmed to worry about the plate size or the way we use our cutlery.

There is part of the theory that has some credence for thinner people, in that the food starts triggering the stomach's equivalent of 'Hotel Full' signs once the food passes through; so eating more slowly triggers those hormones at a point when less food has been eaten. However, whether it works for fat people is more debatable. When I have tried eating a smaller portion, then a couple of hours later I am starving again – but this time the need is even stronger as my body tells me (in no uncertain terms) not to try that daft trick again!

Small is beautiful?

Another theory is that if you eat smaller portions then you 'train' your stomach to shrink in size, so those smaller portions will eventually become more filling. It is another myth. There is a certain elasticity of the stomach which can go both ways, but the concept that you can shrink your stomach through consistently smaller portions is without any basis in fact. Also, the elasticity of the stomach does not control the release of hormones to tell our brain we are full.

Dr. Michael Mosley is a doctor and British television presenter who has advocated the 5:2 diet. By limiting your calorie intake to around 500 a day, for two days per week, the rationale is that you can eat normally for the other five days, or even eat a bit more (by up to 1,000 calories).

I can see how it works for thin people, but as we have seen with the Cabbage Soup diet, it is unrealistic for addressing obesity. Even if we managed 500 calories for two days, the reaction for most Proper Fatties (myself included) over the following five days would be to take in a lot more than 3,500 calories. Fat people are not well-treated by an idea that creates extra urges and desperation; we can do that pretty well already.

Then add in 2018 research at the University of Sao Paolo, Brazil, which suggested intermittent fasting diets can produce molecules in the body called Free Radicals. Studying rats who were made to fast every other day showed decreased body weight, but increased fat tissue plus some damage to insulin-releasing cells in the pancreas. Research leader Ana Bonassa said: "This is the first study to show that, despite weight loss, intermittent fasting diets may actually damage the pancreas and affect insulin function in normal healthy individuals, which could lead to diabetes and serious health issues."

Light as a feather

Another new trend among diets has been weight loss plans which provide low-calorie food options for a period of time, at a price! Jenny Craig is one of the biggest, an American who started her weight loss business in Australia and ended up selling it to multi-national giant Nestle. She offered menu kits and advice; many more have sprung up offering everything from complete meals, and meal replacement, to one-to-one advice.

One is called LighterLife. It has been supported by UK celebrities such as Denise Welch and Pauline Quirke. Birds of a Feather actress Quirke reportedly lost six stone in six months. One of their biggest success stories is Rob Gillett, who was more than 41 stone at one point and managed to lose more than 20 stone on the LighterLife Plan.

Dr. Ellie Cannon revealed on Mail Online a LighterLife phone operator told her that after reaching your weight loss goal, "You can go back to your normal food." The programme recommends a longer-term healthy eating plan designed to keep the weight off, but you know what the phone operator meant!

Most of these schemes emphasise the short-term successes and longer-term statistics are hard to find.

We know from Professor Mann's study that the longer the period of investigation then the higher the percentage of people who regain all the weight and, indeed, the higher the level of overall increase. These figures held true no matter how successful the diet was in the first place and how much weight was lost. I am sure if LighterLife had five, ten, 15 or 20-year figures that showed the vast majority of their clients had fully maintained their weight loss then they would shout it from the rooftops.

Balancing the options

Are there diets which can work? Never mind, for now, the short-term low-calorie options – what about fat-free, low-carb, vegetarian, or vegan approaches?

There are some lessons from the BBC Horizon programme involving twin doctors Chris and Xand Van Tulleken, an unusually accurate example of the comparative effect of very different 'diets' on two identical twins.

Chris went on a high-sugar, low-fat diet. He was allowed to eat things like jelly, bread, pasta, rice, potatoes, cereals, and as much fruit and veg as he liked. If he had wanted to eat an entire bowl of sugar, then he could. He loaded sugar into his coffee to make up for not being able to have milk or cream.

Xand went on a high-fat, low-sugar diet. He could eat meat, cheese, milk, double cream, mayonnaise, burgers, chicken with the skin on, bacon and eggs, but no fruit and very few vegetables. He expected to be craving greens after a few days (my body does not work like that).

Both diets fly in the face of almost all normal diets that you will see in books, magazine, DVDs, and websites, though the high-fat, low-sugar diet has some similarities to the Atkins Diet.

The received wisdom would be that you would put on weight eating as much as you like, the high-sugar diet would be risky in terms of diabetes. If all the people who make millions out of diet advice are right, then these would both be disasters.

Dr. Xand Van Tulleken, on the high-fat, low-sugar diet, lost 3.5 kilograms in a month; that is almost eight pounds and more than half a stone. Dr. Chris Van Tulleken lost a kilogram on his high-sugar, low-fat diet, which is a couple of pounds. For both of them, the weight loss was made up of around 50% body fat and 50% muscle.

It is amazing that they lost weight. Even they admitted it was counter-intuitive. However, there were other important lessons as well. You would have expected the high sugar diet to be bad for diabetes, but actually, the body adjusted to the higher sugar levels, produced more insulin and coped pretty well. However, the low sugar diet led to a reduction of insulin production, and in just a month Xand moved from a safe level of blood glucose to within a fraction of being labelled pre-diabetic. His blood glucose went from 5.1 to 5.9 in that short period, when anything above six is considered pre-diabetic.

In other words, the more successful diet, in weight loss terms, was less successful in terms of diabetes. Typical, there can never be a straightforward answer!

They summed it up as follows. "It is never about one thing. It is always more complicated than that. Always," said Xand. Chris added, "If someone is selling one simple solution to a problem everyone has, then it probably isn't going to work."

Later Xand explained, "All faddish diets, *all faddish diets*, are wrong and misguided – all of them."

Although studying twins is one of the most reliable methods in this area (plus Horizon had the benefit of two doctors with day jobs in medical research) it was still just a one-off for a TV programme.

However, in 2018, a Stanford University randomised clinical trial backed up the findings and went a bit further.[20] Stanford's researchers also discovered there was no real difference between a low-fat or a low-carbohydrate diet – they achieved success over 12 months with groups on both those diets.

While neither diet was better than the other, they did conclude that modifying diet, paying more attention to the content and planning, had a positive impact in itself. In other words, modify your diet but not in a gimmicky way – much as Xand van Tulleken pointed out.

The Lancet published in 2018 a report by scientists from Harvard's School of Public Health and Brigham and Women's Hospital[21] which illustrated life expectancy was lowered by both low and high carbohydrate intake – unsurprisingly a balanced approach of good quality carbohydrates is the way forward.

Vegan and vegetarian diets have become increasingly popular. There are all sorts of arguments which are not really the territory of this book, but from an obesity point of view there are considerations. If you plan your food to a high level, as such a diet necessitates, then you are likely to lose weight whatever the path you follow. In order to avoid long-term health issues, you have to plan the replacement of animal products extremely carefully. For example, 10 ounces of ground beef provides about the same level of important iron as five cups of spinach, both around half the recommended daily intake.

Summary

So diets are expensive, often ineffective, and commonly inefficient. Indeed, diets are the problem, not the solution. The question should not be "how do I lose weight?" – that's obvious. Instead, it should be "why can't many intelligent, committed people lose weight over a long period of time?"

And there's one other problem . . . the obsession with short-term diets blocks the search for solutions which might actually work.

CHAPTER 4

Mindless Exercise

"Exercise is bunk. If you are healthy, you don't need it: if you are sick, you should not take it."

Henry Ford

Thirty minutes of hard exercise per day has been described by the UK's Academy of Medical Royal Colleges as a 'miracle cure' for many things, obesity included. As the Harvard TH Chan School of Public Health puts it: "Being moderately active for at least 30 minutes a day on most days of the week can help lower the risk of chronic disease. But to stay at a healthy weight, or to lose weight, most people will need more physical activity - at least an hour a day - to counteract the effects of increasingly sedentary lifestyles, as well as the strong societal influences that encourage overeating."

For most people that translates roughly into: fat people must be a load of lazy couch potatoes; they just need to get off their fat behinds and go to the gym. It is also a message regularly promoted by the food and drink industry – which should add to any feelings of suspicion.

Of course, exercise is a good thing – something we need to do more of in modern society – and it will be part of any improvement in general health. My point in this chapter is not that exercise is a mistake, but the idea it is a magic cure for obesity is a mistake. There are benefits in exercising enough to increase our heart rates, but they are only inter-linked with obesity; exercise is *not* the answer on its own and, for some, it may be part of the problem.

There is also a real danger of setting the bar too high. How many people in the world do specific physical activity for an hour a day, or hard physical activity for at least half an hour each day? By pushing for such high standards and dismissing anything less, there is a risk of taking away the incentive for people to do anything at all. Activities that do not raise the heart rate will still use calories and can still affect the obesity crisis. By focusing too much on hard exercise, like the Academy of Medical Royal Colleges, we may well be missing a trick. Easy exercise may be a more effective way forward.

So why do the messages in the media put so much emphasis on hard, tough, unpleasant exercise, as opposed to more effective and pleasant alternatives?

Because thin people are leading the debate.

Exercise is often something that comes easy to them; they may even be addicted to it. So much of the comment and societal pressure on overweight people feels as though it's motivated by a desire to see fat people punished, to go through something unpleasant as payback for that extra doughnut. That judgemental approach is shown in magazine and newspaper columns, radio phone-ins, social media, and comments in films. The irony is that you are more likely to have that extra doughnut as a reward after exercise, but that is a different story.

Some people get a 'high' from physical activity; they will get withdrawal symptoms if they do not do enough physical work. Exercise will usually release endorphins, amongst a variety of hormones, which provide some people with a buzz as well as suppressing pain and allowing them to carry on for longer. They activate the opiate centres of the brain; the same receptors that are affected by drugs such as heroin and morphine (and food), so the feelings can be pretty powerful. Not only do you end up wanting to exercise again, but it also hurts less; a perfect double whammy. No wonder it gets to some people, and they train really hard.

Certainly, if you cut out the exercise for someone whose brain rewards exercise with adrenaline and endorphins, then they get edgy – even if it means damaging their body by doing it. I know one person who completed an Iron Man competition (two-mile swim, a 50-mile cycle ride, and a 10-mile run) and who promised himself a well-deserved week off to recover. He was back running four days later, even though (ideally) the body needed more time to recover. There are plenty of others who put their bodies through training that wears out various important parts such as knees and hips; they cannot stop themselves from doing an extra, harmful level of exercise that is unnecessary from a weight control or health point of view.

While many people with a large physical frame will end up being fat, those people who are both big-framed and thin will often achieve that goal through exercise. They have both sides, the exercise genes as well as the fat genes.

There are plenty of studies which show exercise is a good way of keeping thin people thin – but there are also plenty of studies that show it is *not* an effective way of getting fat people thin.

Kevin Allen's research on The Biggest Loser television programme showed that those who did the most exercise were not the ones to lose the most weight, though exercise after the programme finished was significant in those who kept weight down. There are also many reviews which show that exercise has a far lower impact on weight loss than other efforts. The National Weight Control Registry, the biggest such study established in 1994 by scientists from Brown University and the University of Colorado, has exercise as just one of many common factors in sustained weight loss. One of the key studies was by the University of Louisiana[22] which put hundreds of women on varying exercise regimes for six months, plus a group which did no extra exercise. The results were level across the groups, showing the varying levels of exercise had not helped people lose weight. It is categorically not as simple as 'calories in versus calories out.'

Some would argue that less physical activity is a central cause of the obesity epidemic over the last 40 years. Although there is a lack of appropriate, widespread, large-scale research over the whole period, there is research which knocks down any link between obesity rates and decreased exercise. A Minnesota Heart Survey between 1980 and 2002 found little or no change to the amount of time spent per week in physical activity. Over essentially the same period, from 1980 to 2000, US adult obesity is calculated to have doubled; childhood obesity has tripled.[23]

The US Behavioural Risk Factor Surveillance System found physical activity actually went up around 5% in the US between 1990 and 2007, both in terms of more people doing vigorous physical activity and more taking part in some physical activity. Quite simply, the research confirms a lack of exercise cannot be the explanation for the rise in obesity over the last 40 years.

Drs. Ronald Iannotti and Jing Wang, of the Eunice Kennedy Shriver National Institute of Child Health and Human Development, published a report in 2013 on the behaviour of US adolescents between 2001 and 2009. They showed improvements in diet and exercise while obesity rates continued to rise. They concluded, "These patterns suggest that public health efforts to improve the obesity-related behaviours of US adolescents may be having some success. However, alternative explanations for the increase in BMI over the same period need to be considered."

Some blame current trends of video games, TV, social media and the internet as factors, but increased obesity is an issue that pre-dates these technological developments. In the period when Netflix, Amazon, Xbox, PlayStation and the rest have taken hold, we have seen a continuation or – in some advanced countries – a slowing down of the rise in obesity rates.

There is Kevin Allen's research into the metabolic rate of The Biggest Loser participants changing to compensate for the reduced calories intake and increased exercise. There is also a Laval University, Quebec, report published in Obesity Research in 1994 which showed, through studies on overweight twins, that an increased level of exercise produced only slight weight loss and much, much less than would have been expected under the 'calories in, calories out' model. The research was part of the long-running Quebec Family Study which started in 1978 and continues to have a major impact on the obesity debate to this day.

None of which takes away from the wider benefits of exercise. For some people it is like taking heroin, but with generally beneficial side effects instead of damaging ones. It sounds perfect; I wish I felt that way. Unfortunately, I can't say I have ever felt that buzz, second wind, or sense of elation from exercise. Not once.

I've had some odd looks when I say that, but it never entered my head that someone could feel euphoric at the end of training until I was asked why I wasn't inspired by it. People walk away from training talking about it being a 'good' or 'great' session. I might think it an effective or necessary session, at best, but never good or great!

Buzz off

Dopamine is one of the main reward systems of the human body; it makes us feel good about things like alcohol, nicotine, caffeine, and various other drugs (including cocaine, marijuana, and heroin).

A person's brain is used to a particular level of dopamine activity and when this level increases, a compensation process kicks in (in order to moderate intake or behaviour) which sees the brain reduce the number of receptors in order to get dopamine back down to earlier levels. In doing so, a person looking for more of the feel-good effect needs to take more of something to get the same uplift from fewer receptors. Medical journal The Lancet revealed that obese people have a reduced number of dopamine receptors (whilst food-seeking increases dopamine levels by around 50%). In other words, the brain feels good when seeking and eating food, but because there are fewer receptors, the signals to the body that 'enough is enough' get impaired, and we keep going when others are happy to stop.

There is a debate over whether that difference in the brain is caused by the act of overeating or is, itself, the cause of overeating. No-one wants to let fat people off the hook, so there are plenty who favour the first theory. I favour the second. There is plenty of evidence that our brains are affected by genetics, time in the womb, and early life; less so by non-specific events in adulthood such as over-eating.

Exercise brings wide-ranging health benefits, helps you carry out other activities in greater comfort, and can help in terms of friendships and relationships. I am a big believer in sport and, by extension, exercise.

There is a risk for the majority though. There is a natural feeling that by exercising you have earned the right to eat or drink something nice. The body craves recovery and pushes for extra nutrition to compensate for the resources used up in exercise.

Well, you need to run about four to five miles to 'earn' a bar of chocolate, whilst you would need to walk six or seven miles for the same effect. A single MacDonald's small hamburger would mean running two miles at a good pace, or walking three, while a Big Tasty with Bacon and medium fries would need a ten-mile run or 15-mile walk before you could 'earn' it. I used to do the rowing machine for an hour; the machine would tell me I had worked off around 400-600 calories (I'm not sure I ever fully believed it, but that's a different point) – less than the two cheeseburgers I felt I had earned as a result. One was an hour of effort, without any mental stimulus or buzz, while the other took less than five minutes with plenty of mental reward. The maths did not stack up in my favour!

All walk, no play

There is plenty of evidence to show we 'reward' ourselves for doing exercise. Research also shows that if we exercise three times a week, for example, we tend to do less the rest of the time because we feel we have earned a chance to relax. Not only do we do less on the days we have been to the gym, but we also tend to do less on the other days as well, hence the reason we do less overall.

Put all that together over a week and three reasonable gym sessions – say expending 500 calories per time – and it totals just 1500 calories. Seven days of getting up to make the tea, walking the dog, being the one who nips out to the shop, walking instead of driving (or, taking the bike!) or all the other small ways of using a few calories here and there, would use many thousands of calories.

It may well be different in men and women. 2013 University of Iran research discovered women compensated for 23% of their energy deficit through eating afterwards, while men actually ate less than normal after a gym session.[24]

The London School of Economics did a report which showed how regular brisk walking was better for weight loss than going to the gym. Of course, they had to include a bit of fat-bashing – moaning about the obesity crisis – before arriving at a statement of the obvious.

Walking is attainable, even for fat people. Lycra-swamped gyms are not exactly the place where a fat person can feel most at home.

Blockhead

In our Fat Class, one lady was praised continually for going to water aerobics once a week. A good thing to do, naturally, for social as well as physical reasons, but hardly the panacea it was being portrayed as. In another session, she responded to one of my comments by asking if she should walk around the block first thing every morning. The reply from the instructor was that it would do nothing to build up her heart rate and lose weight, so stick to the aqua-aerobics once a week.

It was a frustratingly rubbish answer. Of course, she should walk around the block every morning! Of course, that would make more of a difference. Even if it was just 400 yards around the block, that would be a couple of miles a week, could lead to longer walks, more often, and almost certainly more calories lost per week than one water aerobics session. Walking does not rule out weekly aqua-aerobics, but walking is much more likely to be something you can turn into a long-term, regular habit with all the benefits that would involve.

Finding time for an hour's hard exercise a day, something which will generally take up to two hours (when travel and changing are taken into account) is not always easy. Shorter, easier things we can do should be the focus, rather than all or nothing.

In terms of a hard one-hour training session in a gym, studies show it is an equivalent calorie burn to standing up for three hours. Certainly, tests show that a waiter or waitress will use the same number of calories over a busy lunchtime of serving customers. I would call it the dog walking effect. People who regularly walk their dogs are rarely badly overweight, no matter what other bad habits they may have in their lives. There is a drip, drip, drip effect; a regular use of calories. They may not walk that far, but they do it a couple of times a day and are standing up the whole time as well.

Above all, exercising to lose weight is not a straightforward trade-off. It has been shown the human body is capable of adapting to extreme exercise without using extra calories. Studies on the super-active Hadza tribe in Tanzania show their bodies compensate to use the same number of calories per day as a typical Westerner, despite their non-stop busy-ness as one of the last remaining hunter-gather tribes on the planet.[25]

There is another simple way to avoid putting on weight – fidgeting. According to the Mayo Clinic in 2010, an academic medical centre in Minnesota, lean people have trouble holding still; they pace and fidget for at least two hours a day while overweight people just sit. They calculated the difference at 350 calories a day. They give the credit for such useful activity to genetically-determined levels of brain hormones. It was rigorous research based on volunteers wearing underwear with special sensors, while a team of 150 researchers ploughed through the resulting 25 million pieces of data.

As part of the study, they found activity levels were unaffected by weight changes in the group. This emphasised the genetic link, rather than a weight-related choice.

Unfortunately, this knowledge is not much use to anyone trying to combat obesity. It has to be natural and subconscious. I have tried to fidget, but can only do so when I concentrate on fidgeting – it simply isn't possible to do that for two hours a day.

The broad point, however, is that using calories is not all about hard physical exercise. Using our brains takes up calories, even when we are not thinking hard. A resting brain will use around 250 calories a day, about the same as a half-hour training session, and more as it gets used. People who watch a horror movie use more calories than someone watching a rom-com, just because our brains are more stimulated.

It means that standing in front of a mirror thinking you look fat, uses up calories! At least that is some consolation.

So, while exercise is a good thing in its own right, and is definitely an important *part* of the fight against obesity, it works best in preventing weight gain rather than losing it. It helps thin people, mostly, for four reasons:

1. They probably get more of a mental reward from doing it, so will carry on.

2. They are probably fit enough to work harder and go further, using more calories.

3. Their 'treat' will be a biscuit; a fat person's 'treat' will be a packet of biscuits.

4. The fatter you are, the harder the exercise. Your size means you use more calories per effort, but will find it harder to keep going.

So, the gym, training sessions, personal trainers – these are all thin people's solutions. They are harder for fat people to achieve and may well, paradoxically, have a negative impact on calorie intake and general activity.

More dangerously, the exercise message can be counter-productive. It can distract people from more achievable activities. The more emphasis put on an hour of hard exercise every day – the more that everything else is dismissed, and the more that obesity rates will rise.

Doing a little more every day will have an impact that is more achievable, and more attainable, for many fat people than an hour of hard exercise.

The fat person's answer is to increase activity as much as possible, but in a sustainable way. It is all the classic things:

Walk the dog.

Park further from work or get off a stop early and walk.

Do the shopping and park further away in the car park.

Do small, regular shops with a basket, not a huge, weekly shop with a trolley.

Walk around the block every morning.

Take the stairs instead of the lift, always (unless you're late for a job interview on the 22nd floor).

Go for regular walks or bike rides – better to do fewer, regularly, than target a huge challenge which proves off-putting.

These are just some examples; there are plenty of self-help books which will give much longer lists of recommendations – some of them are even good ideas. Will all that help you lose weight? Well, it might help a little.

Oh, and train if you can. It might not help your weight, but it's good for you in all sorts of other ways. But while exercise is good, the concentration on it from a weight loss point of view is bad. It may even be a little more sinister than that.

As a group of international scientists wrote in the British Journal of Sports Medicine in 2015 [26] "It is time to bust the myth of physical inactivity and obesity, you cannot outrun a bad diet."

They explain, "members of the public are drowned by an unhelpful message about maintaining a 'healthy weight' through calorie counting, and many still wrongly believe that obesity is entirely due to lack of exercise. This false perception is rooted in the Food Industry's Public Relations machinery, which uses tactics chillingly similar to those of big tobacco. The tobacco industry successfully stalled government intervention for 50 years starting from when the first links between smoking and lung cancer were published. This sabotage was achieved using a 'corporate playbook' of denial, doubt and confusing the public

"Coca-Cola, who spent $3.3 billion on advertising in 2013, pushes a message that 'all calories count'; they associate their products with sport, suggesting it is ok to consume their drinks as long as you exercise. However, science tells us this is misleading and wrong. It is where the calories come from that is crucial. Sugar calories promote fat storage and hunger. Fat calories induce fullness or 'satiation'.

"It is time to wind back the harms caused by the junk food industry's public relations machinery. Let us bust the myth of physical inactivity and obesity. You cannot outrun a bad diet."

CHAPTER 5

So Why Are We Fat?

"My doctor told me to stop having intimate dinners for four. Unless there are three other people."

Orson Welles

Former England international rugby player Brian Moore wrote a fascinating book which detailed incidents of abuse he suffered as a child and the battles with depression he had as an adult, probably as a direct result. He came up with a very good analogy, describing depression as his inner 'Gollum' after the character in Lord of the Rings who skulks in the shadows, part friend, part enemy. Gollum is not one of the Fellowship of the Ring, but he's a key player; never far away, persuasive and manipulative.

Moore felt his depression was not really part of him, but a separate force within his body which he could not control. It appeared without bidding; it drove him to think things he did not want to think, to feel and do things he did not want to do. It was a bit like the Tom and Jerry cartoons, with the devil on one shoulder and the angel on the other.

If I take the Gollum analogy and run with it, then I would talk about the inner Jolly Green Giant of fat people. Just like depression, there is an inner 'being' which influences our behaviour, our bodies, in ways we do not like or want, like an addiction we cannot control.

Many will knock the idea of comparing something as serious as depression with obesity, but it would not have seemed strange a few years ago when depression was often dismissed. For years, there was a gap between the understanding of mental health professionals and the 'pull yourself together' view of public opinion, similar to the growing scientific explanations of obesity versus the 'eat less, move more' message.

We have only recently begun to accept depression is more than something to 'snap out of' – thanks partly to a number of celebrities, such as Moore, who have been prepared to come forward and talk about their own struggles. To quote the heartfelt comment from Carrie Carlisle, the wife of former professional footballer Clarke Carlisle who suffers from life-threatening depression, who told the BBC, "If I could go back and change anything it would be to stop using myself, my own mental framework, as a reference. It is a huge mistake."

Depression's chemical imbalance in the brain has many similarities with obesity and a variety of triggers, both social and genetic. There are elements of modern life which seem to increase the numbers suffering from depression, just as obesity has increased dramatically in the last 40 years. As psychotherapist Mel Schwartz asked in Psychology Today, in 2012, "Is our society manufacturing depressed people?" With more than 20% of the American population experiencing at least one episode of clinical depression (estimates have gone up slightly since 2012), he argues that modern society is not only to blame but that "under certain circumstances, it makes sense to be depressed."

While changes in society are clearly one factor I will return to, another is that there is a significant genetic element in both depression and obesity. A 2008 study by University College and King's College, London, published in the American Journal of Clinical Nutrition[27] set out to quantify the genetic element of being overweight. "Body mass index (BMI) has been shown to be highly heritable, but most studies were carried out in cohorts born before the onset of the obesity epidemic," they stated.

The researchers studied British twins between the ages of 8-11 – both identical and non-identical – so the social influences of parenting, schooling, and environment are highly similar, making the results more reliable than if the tests had been carried out on adults. The researchers also studied weight gain around the waist as well as general BMI, which is a fairer measure. There were much greater differences in weight and waist size in the non-identical twins compared to identical twins, showing that different genetics were a key element. In conclusion, the study estimated that genetics accounted for around 75% of both obesity and weight gain around the waist.

"These results indicate that adiposity (fat) in preadolescent children born since the onset of the obesity epidemic is highly heritable. The heritability of BMI in this sample (77%) is at the higher end of results obtained with large adult samples," explained the researchers, who downplayed the importance of the social approaches.

"The fact that siblings' experience of being served similar food, being given the same options for television viewing and active outdoor play, seeing the same behaviours modelled by parents, and going to the same school does not make siblings more similar is a challenge for etiologic models that highlight the home environment as the root cause of obesity."

It is an argument taken further by Robert Plomin, an American psychologist and geneticist based at King's College, London. He argues that genetics are responsible for all sorts of behaviours and achievements previously credited to the environment. With advances in genetic studies, it is an area we know more and more about.

Plomin used the example of depression in a Guardian interview about his book Blueprint: How DNA Makes Us Who We Are. If we find genetic differences between large enough groups of depressed and non-depressed people, then the more of those differences that occur in someone, the more likely they are to be depressed. He argues it is about probability, rather than illness. "That means you can't cure a disorder because there is no disorder," he says. Being depressed, in this case, is about DNA rather than choice.

Simply put, there is much, much more to obesity than blaming lifestyle and parenting.

It's about the brain, stupid

Bill Clinton's 1992 US presidential campaign coined the phrase, 'It's the economy, stupid' when it came to the main motivation for people voting. I would paraphrase it to say, 'It's about the brain, stupid,' when it comes to the main motivation for people eating.

Dr. Chris van Tulleken and Prof. Tanya Byron teamed up with scientists from Oxford and Cambridge universities for the BBC TV programme What's the Right Diet for You? in which they measured stomach hormones as a way of predicting how much food people would eat from a Tapas bar of rotating and freely available food. They were accurate in their predictions; those with the highest hormone levels ate the most. Then the shock came when they boasted how no-one had ever done this experiment before.

$800 million dollars of research in the US alone and no-one had ever followed the links between hormones and appetite that closely before? You couldn't make it up.

The human brain is the most complicated organism or 'invention' on the planet; we like to compare it to a supercomputer. While computers may be superior in terms of memory and sifting through large amounts of information, in many ways, the human brain is way more advanced than any computer yet conceived (in the real world anyway). Yet, that incredible complexity of structure, individual development, and hormones means there are so many ways we can be different from each other.

While we do not have a deep understanding or wholly reliable treatment for conditions such as depression or Post Traumatic Stress Disorder (or over-eating), we do have a greater realisation that the balance of the brain has changed in people with depression or PTSD; they have hormonal reasons for not thinking the same way as many others – even others going through a similar situation.

Back in World War I, 306 British soldiers were executed because they were suffering from 'shell shock' and would not go back to the front to fight. It's a misunderstanding summed up by the case of British soldier Harry Farr who was shot for cowardice in 1916 after a series of incidents we would clearly diagnose now as PTSD. Yet, this 'coward' was brave enough to face his firing squad without the blindfold he was offered.[28] 100 years on, we understand the reality of PTSD: the genuine, physical changes to the brain caused by a sudden and dramatic event such as war or a terrorist attack.

Essentially PTSD is an overreaction, triggered by the memory of a former situation which was really bad. The amygdala section of the brain is more easily prompted to put out danger signs to the rest of the brain, prompting over-the-top behaviour or fear in relatively 'normal' situations. It is a hormonal response, and the fact that not everyone reacts in the same way does not make it less real for those who do.

We now understand those people with 'shell shock' needed sympathetic treatment, not execution.

In turn, we know that depression can be influenced by genetics, various developments while we are in the womb, and shock events in life. For instance, people whose mothers smoked during pregnancy are more likely to get depressed and have above average aggression levels.

Self-harm is an area of increasing concern. It seems hard to believe anyone would use pain as a way of dealing with depression. However, thanks to listening compassionately to self-harmers, we now understand it is about being in control of the pain, to make up for other areas where they lack control. Pain releases various hormones that help combat some people's depression in the short-term.

Treating depression is an uncertain science, and there is still some stigma attached, but at least we are making progress thanks to sympathetic research and an increased desire to understand. We treat depression with drugs, sometimes, to restore the brain's chemical balance. It is an interesting starting point; the problem is that the brain is so complex we have no certain way of being able to administer drugs that will work and also no certainty about possible side effects.

We are learning about how exercise, meditation, and cold water swimming (amongst other physical activities), can help the body to produce the hormones needed to counter depression more naturally.

And, ironically for people who are depressed about their weight, there is truth in the phrase 'comfort eating'. Eating fatty and sugary foods can trigger the reward system of the brain and help to combat depression.

Fat Head

Depression, PTSD, all very interesting; but some will ask what they have to do with people eating too much. Well, the point is we do not have a separate, more controllable, section of the brain that deals with our urges to eat. The brain chemistry of over-eating is much more like depression, PTSD, or addiction than many people like to think. The more we can understand all these areas, the more we can understand each of them.

It's funny, being called a Fat Head is an insult – it is about being stupid, doing something ridiculous. However, there may be only one part of the body which does not get overweight, and that is the brain (cheeks and jowls, maybe, brain no). In fact, there is research that obesity makes the brain smaller, possibly some 8% smaller for the truly obese and 4% smaller for the merely overweight. There are some links, then, to increased risks of Alzheimer's and dementia because memory areas are affected.

The phrase Fat Head makes sense in a different way to me – we are fat because of what goes on in our heads. We need to delve a little deeper into the workings of our brains if we are to understand obesity. The key is understanding just what makes us eat more than we want or need.

For those who still need persuading, I racked my brain (non-fatty version) trying to think of something to show how little control over our brain's hormones we sometimes have. I will start with a really simple example.

Everyone at some time or another has struggled to get to sleep. We know we really need to get to sleep, we need a full night's sleep to be on top form for the following day's competition, interview, work, or task – whatever it may be. This is not a case of staying up partying, or finishing some chore; we are in bed, and we want to go to sleep.

But we can't.

We toss and turn, trying to get comfortable. Just when we want our minds to empty, they go into overdrive. We plan situations in detail, whether real or imagined. We turn things over, we think of alternatives. In fact, we do pretty much everything other than the one thing we really want to do. Try willpower if you like, really try to go to sleep; if anything, it's counter-productive.

Our conscious minds have no doubt about what we should be doing and what we want to be doing, but our conscious minds have no power. The more we think we really need to go to sleep, the less likely we are to be able to do it. We deploy habits, routines, and expectations – things which will usually trigger sleep hormones – but, once the brain is alert, there is not a lot we can do.

Sleep is an interesting example in a lot of ways. Firstly, we do not really need to do it at all in terms of bodily recovery. The body regenerates in some minor ways, it relaxes obviously, and the brain gets a chance to file some of that day's information, but none of these are essential to our survival as a species in modern society.

Sleep is really just a way of hitting the pause button in our lives until we are ready for the world and the world is a safer place for us. Some other animals are better prepared for the dark, so being awake at the same time as these potential predators was dangerous for our ancestors. Sleeping in the dark and being awake in the light is something that has developed over millions of years through our evolution rather than something we need physically. Something our bodies grew to rely on.

The body of every animal needs some sort of rest but, from a physical recovery point of view, it can be pretty brief and varied according to the circumstances. Different animals sleep in different ways and at different times. Some hibernate over the winter when foodstuffs are scarce; fish have periods when they reduce their metabolism and brain activity, but it is not sleep as we know it. Sharks do not go into a deep sleep like humans; it seems likely their swimming is co-ordinated from the spine rather than the brain so they can do what is called 'sleep-swimming.' Koalas are pretty safe asleep up in their trees, so they sleep for around 90% of the time and have a lifestyle and food supply that helps them do just that. Sleep just happens to be another thing we have in common with most mammals.

Our body clock and circadian rhythms (natural sleep patterns) have become so important that a lack of sleep has even been credited as one indicator of obesity – maybe because it gives us more time to eat!

Sleep is brought on by various hormones being released, in particular, melatonin. The signals sent to other parts of the brain make us feel sleepy or wide awake. Light triggers a nerve at the back of the eye's retina which leads to the hypothalamus, which in turn releases other chemicals around the brain to wake us. When we cannot get to sleep, it is a combination of melatonin not being released, or the release of other chemicals stimulating the brain and overriding that effect.

Sometimes there can be an extreme imbalance, such as narcolepsy when people find it difficult to stay awake through the day. We do not choose to be narcoleptic, and no amount of willpower will make a difference. To show the overlapping nature of these areas, narcolepsy drugs are sometimes prescribed for depression.

At the other end of the scale, some people can get away with very little sleep, two to three hours a night; in fact, they find it generally physically impossible to sleep the eight hours that would be the desire of the average person. Former British Prime Minister Margaret Thatcher was one of those people who could only sleep four hours each night. Some Thatcher fans think that is an example of her great determination, but that is pretty unlikely. Studies on families who do not need much sleep have revealed genetic variations are the cause. University of California, San Francisco, Professor Ying-Hui Fu discovered the mutation in gene DEC2 in 2009, backed up in 2018 studies on mice, in people who naturally woke early. Researchers at the Centre for Applied Genomics in Philadelphia narrowed it down further to the p.Tyr362 mutation of the DEC2 gene in 2014, after studies on twins who slept different lengths of time.

Mind control

Other areas which are controlled by the hypothalamus include body temperature, parental attachments, and thirst. A man called Wim Hof can control his body temperature to the extent that he can stay in icy water for two hours and keep his core body temperature normal. So can practitioners of the ancient art of Tummo in Tibet.

And the hypothalamus controls hunger.

Dutch doctor Dick Swaab's 2014 book We Are Our Brains makes the case that genetics are obviously the starting point, the development of the brain in the womb is the next crucial stage, and then there are factors in the early years of life when the brain is still developing and growing which also shape who we are.

He explains clearly that areas such as aggression, our propensity for depression or other mental illnesses, gender identity, and sexual orientation, are among the things that are pretty much set in stone before we go to primary school. Whatever happens afterwards just brings out these pre-programmed traits, in a massive range of areas where we think we have greater control.

To take one tiny example, "Men with a tiny variation in a DNA building block for the vasopressin receptor (the protein that receives vasopressin's message in the brain) are twice as likely to experience marital difficulties and divorce and twice as likely to be unfaithful," he writes. Vasopressin is a hormone that plays an important role in social behaviour, sexual motivation, and pair bonding. So, something we think of as a lifestyle choice is actually influenced by our hormonal make-up.

He is also very clear about obesity, which he acknowledges is a growing problem (no pun intended). "That so many people are fat isn't just due to a lack of self-control. Predisposition is certainly a factor. Obesity has a strong genetic component. Studies of twins, adopted children, and families, indicate that around 80 percent of the variation in body weight is determined by genetic factors," he writes.

He puts into technical language things that fat people know instinctively, but it's still nice to get a scientific explanation that doesn't mention 'willpower' or 'lifestyle choice'. Except in downplaying them.

"Normally, the hypothalamus registers how much fat our body has stored by measuring the amount of leptin, a hormone produced by fat tissue. If there are mutations in the leptin gene or the leptin receptor, the hypothalamus will conclude that there's no fat tissue and continually prompt you to eat, resulting in morbid obesity."

As we find out more about the way the brain works – and the way these processes control us – we begin to understand more.

Depression, the mother smoking during pregnancy, and trauma during the birth itself and/or early life of the baby, are among the factors that can often release the hormones which cause obesity. Over-feeding the baby or the mother being overweight during pregnancy can also increase the chances.

It can work the other way too. Fascinatingly, mothers who were pregnant in the Netherlands during a famine in the final months of World War II, caused by the Nazi occupation, gave birth to children who had higher rates of obesity. This particular incident has led to further research that may help to explain why so many people are fat in the modern era.

A team of epigeneticists from Israel and America looked at how the body responds to starvation through the generations. They discovered the 'memory of starvation' can get passed down in our DNA, which works through messages carried by ribonucleic acid (RNA). Dr. Oded Rechavi, explained in Medicine Daily, "To the best of our knowledge, our paper provides the first concrete evidence that it's enough to simply experience a particular environment – in this case, an environment without food – for small RNA inheritance and RNA interference to ensue."

The researchers started by examining the Nazi blockade of the Western Netherlands, but got hands-on in the laboratory and used worms to see the effect in action. The research showed the DNA linked to starvation could go through at least three generations. Oddly, the use of marijuana is another desire which can be handed down through the generations.

As a side note, Swaab bemoans the fact that many victims of anorexia nervosa will not allow their brains to be studied for medical research after they die, because they believe the myth that anorexia is just a question of willpower rather than a chemical balance. By holding that viewpoint, Dr. Swaab says, they are hindering the speed with which we can understand the problem. They have given into the same bullying that fat people suffer; that their problems are caused by mental weakness rather than physical factors. Indeed, there is evidence that a propensity to be anorexic is also genetic.

Of course, anorexia is the opposite end of the scale to over-eating, but the way the brain's hormones drive bad decisions is identical. We know abnormalities of the hypothalamus often lead to eating disorders at both ends of the spectrum. If anorexia is one end, then Prader-Willi Syndrome is the other extreme where children can never eat enough, thanks to a defective hypothalamus. There is even the condition called Lipoma where areas of fat grow into lumps, much as cancer grows. People think, wrongly, that because it is fat, it can be addressed by diet or exercise, though the cause is genetic damage to the control of cell division. It can affect anyone but predominantly affects women over the age of 50.

The biology of the brain

The biology of the brain is every bit as important to the explanation of obesity as the biology of the rest of the body. What we think of as free decisions can actually be as pre-programmed as any other biological reaction. While the sleep comparison is a little off the wall, the general idea of having much less control over our actions than we imagine is one I believe proved by the curious combination of scientists and magicians!

Magicians, throughout history, have presented the gap between our perception of choice and the psychological reality as something mystical. They use that psychological knowledge as magic, ways of 'forcing' (to use the magicians' term) a member of the public to pick a particular card, to tie in a supposedly free choice with a pre-prepared prediction by the magician.

I enjoyed one trick by British illusionist Katherine Mills when she got a bingo caller to make up his own numbers rather than drawing them by random, while all the people playing the game were allowed independently to choose their numbers as well. The result was that every single person in the room won at the same time, as it turned out Mills had predicted. Everyone would have felt they were making an individual, free choice, but for the trick to work a whole room of people would have been subtly influenced into picking the same numbers. It is all a curious overlap between science and mystique – which capitalizes on our naivety!

As an example closer to home, supermarkets are beginning to spend money on cognitive neuroscience experts to tell the difference between what we say we want and what we actually buy.

Retail experts have found this evidence to be much more accurate than focus groups, where shoppers talk about what they want. We say one thing, but often do another, and it is commercially important to understand that difference. For example, we may say we like informative labels, but we are drawn to buy those products with simple, uncluttered labels. The results show how we react to the colour of packaging, item placement in shops, the amount and type of information on packets; all these things appeal to our subconscious rather than conscious minds.

These approaches have also been used for a long time, either consciously or unconsciously, in marketing. Almost all the major brands of breakfast cereals have a cartoon character on the front of the packaging, with the eyes looking slightly down so the angle will meet the stare of a child from pretty much any shelf other than the bottom one. The overlap between 'magic' and marketing can be surprisingly big.

Another area where our decision-making processes play a lesser part than you may imagine, is in falling in love. Many people will know the feelings – being able to think of little other than the person you love, focussing on them all the time, feeling different, happier, when they are around. Increasingly we understand that those decisions about who we fall in love with are the results of chemical reactions to particular people. We do not fall in love with everyone we fancy physically or get on with as friends; in the end, the evolutionary process moves us towards finding someone who is an appropriate biological match – or at least that's the aim. Sometimes that means someone who seems inappropriate in many other ways.

That may not be the stuff of poetry or songs, but it is the neuroscientific reality. 'Shall I compare thee to a summer's day? Thou art more lovely and a better biological match' does not quite have the same ring about it. Or 'A feeling of evolutionary compatibility is all around me' would not be a Number One hit song– you get the general idea.

So what has all this got to do with eating?

So, all very interesting, you might say, but what is the relevance to obesity? As we understand the brain a little better, I begin to understand why I make bad decisions which give no great pleasure – and which lead me to being overweight.

Like not being able to get to sleep, I feel desires for food I do not want. Just as a magician can manipulate us to make a trick work, so the food retailers and manufacturers spend a fortune on persuading us to buy stuff that is bad for us.

So if you started this book thinking that obesity is a matter of willpower and dieting, has your position shifted? Do you have any sympathy for those children born in the Western Netherlands in 1944 after a period of starvation by the occupying Nazi Germans? What about children born to fat parents, who are also genetically likely to be fat? The point is that a similar hormonal framework exists for most groups of fat people in the world.

Despite all this evidence from extremely learned people, we still find it hard to ignore our own mental framework as a reference point, no matter how much of a mistake that may be. It is hard to understand that level of desperation for food if you do not feel it yourself. If you are a thin person reading this, then you may still think you have a right to say that fat people lack your self-control. So, finally, let's look at situations where hormones have probably overridden your self-control. Have you:

- Been angry when a rational analysis of the situation would have dictated a calmer reaction.
- Been scared of something that is not really that scary.
- Tried things you shouldn't have, as a teenager.
- Argued with your parents when they're right.
- Been overprotective with your children.
- Been a stroppy brother/sister.
- Exercised because you want to.
- Enjoyed a roller coaster/amusement park ride/parachute jump/bungee jump or something even more extreme.
- Been in love or lust.

The list can go on and on but, basically, if you have ever done anything that is not based on a full flowchart of rational analysis, then you have given in to your hormonal and instinctive urges at some time or another. We all do. We have been programmed that way over millions of years. Those hormonal urges have allowed mankind to live, thrive, and survive.

We all give in to something; it reinforces the idea you are just lucky if your urges take you in a different direction.

One thing is certain, though, as many commentators have pointed out **– in the battle of mind over metabolism, it is the latter which wins every time.**

CHAPTER 6

Is Obesity An Addiction?

"Don't ever think you're better than a drug addict, because your brain works the same as theirs. You have the same circuits. And drugs would affect your brain in the same way it affects theirs."

Oliver Markus

If we are beginning to know what obesity is not, we still have to define what it is. Is it a disease or a choice? A compulsion or a desire? A need or a craving? An addiction or a habit?

First, the 'A' word. Can we call over-eating an addiction? There are plenty who still scoff at the idea (remember three-quarters of those taking part in the biggest US survey believe obese people just need to show more willpower). Plenty believe calling obesity an addiction or a disease is just politically-correct nonsense to give fat people an excuse. 'Honestly, soon we won't be allowed to call fat people fat, they'll be width-challenged!'

So let's look at the facts.

The word 'addiction' comes from the Latin 'addictio' meaning a giving over or surrender. The dictionary definition is the 'state of being enslaved to a habit or practice or to something that is psychologically or physically habit-forming, such as narcotics, to such an extent that its cessation causes severe trauma.'

Author Tony Schwartz describes addiction as "the relentless pull to a substance or an activity that becomes so compulsive it ultimately interferes with everyday life."

Increasingly, scientists are becoming able to define addiction in terms of the anatomical changes in the brain; the way messages are carried and received – or not – across the brain's complicated processes. "In a sense, addiction is a pathological form of learning," explained Antonello Bonci, a neurologist at the National Institute on Drug Abuse, to National Geographic in 2017.

Addiction hijacks or changes an individual's neural processes, which also helps to explain why it's easy to journey from one addiction to another – indeed, it's why we talk about pathway or gateway drugs. We accept the urges for sex or drugs are strong and hard to control, but somehow the body's need for food is downgraded to a mere craving. However, we also know that food in general – and some argue sugar in particular – triggers the same brain reaction as sex or drugs, the same pleasure hormones in the same part of the brain.

In 1982, Scientific American published an article arguing that cocaine was no more addictive than eating crisps. At the time, they were widely criticised for making cocaine addiction sound so weak. Now, many experts believe they were right to make the comparison – because we understand the addictive power of eating is so strong.

Researchers at the University of Bordeaux in France found that an amazing 94 percent of rats would choose sugar over cocaine – even those that had been made to be addicted to cocaine beforehand.

The Icahn School of Medicine in Mount Sinai, Israel, has estimated that refined sugar in processed food is eight times more addictive than cocaine. Pizzas are the most addictive food of all, explained Dr. Nicole Avena from the School, thanks to the sugar included in the tomato sauce in particular. Chips, cookies, and ice cream are the next most addictive foodstuffs. Just in case you're wondering, cucumbers, carrots and green beans are the least addictive foods.

A separate study by Connecticut College's neuroscience department suggested that Oreos are as addictive as cocaine and heroin (or, to be more accurate, morphine as a heroin derivative).

Fat rats

The Scripps Research Institute in Jupiter, Florida, experimented with three groups of rats. One was given normal rat food, the second was allowed sweet and fatty foods for just one hour a day, and the third group was offered a 24-hour diet of sweet and fatty foods.

The first group of rats carried on as normal, the second started eating only during that one hour binge each day even though normal food was available all the time, but the most important discovery related to the third group. The 'extended access' group starting eating twice as many calories as the others and became obese. More than that, their brains' reward centres changed so it became harder and harder for them to feel pleasure – an effect which is typical in addiction. The more weight they gained, the worse that effect got.

These rats needed to eat more and more before the internal 'House Full' signs came up. Study author Paul Kenny, an Associate Professor of Neuroscience at Scripps, says the reaction was, "very similar to what we see with animals that use cocaine and heroin."

An international team, including the University of Edinburgh, argued in 2016 that eating is an addiction, but that no particular foods – such as fats and sugars – are more addictive than others. As such, they argue, it is a behavioural addiction like gambling, rather than a substance addiction, like drugs. Either way, they believe we should look at how to classify over-eating as a "mental disorder."

So, what does it mean if you are addicted to something?

Let's start with smoking where there are huge health hazards – even worse than being overweight! That first puff gives your brain a burst of various dopamines, the brain's rewards chemicals. Most cigarette manufacturers also use ammonia and other chemicals to boost the addictive effectiveness of their product. Once you have first experienced smoking, you want to experience it again and again, but here's the catch – each time you experience it, your body gets that little bit more used to the effects. As such, you need more and more to experience the same burst of brain chemicals as that first puff.

The same happens with recreational drugs; they fire the reward system in the brain with some drugs stimulates the spiritual parts of the brain to the extent that religious fervour and drug taking can actually be a very similar experience. Again, the brain wants more and more. Some people can stop before it is too late, but some cannot. Once again, our bodies plainly react differently.

Addictive personality

It seems impossible to argue against eating as an addiction under any of those definitions. We are giving over, surrendering, enslaved, it is habit-forming – while the cessation of eating certainly causes severe trauma!

The next question is this: is addiction a disease or a moral issue? Increasingly the scientific community seems clear about the answer. In 2016, the US Surgeon General, Vivek Murthy, released a report into Alcohol, Drugs, and Health. He said, "For far too long, too many in our country have viewed addiction as a moral failing. This unfortunate stigma has created an added burden of shame that has made people with substance use disorders less likely to come forward and seek help. It has also made it more challenging to marshal the necessary investments in prevention and treatment. We must help everyone see that addiction is not a character flaw – it is a chronic illness that we must approach with the same skill and compassion with which we approach heart disease, diabetes, and cancer."

We are developing a greater understanding that some people have a genetic predisposition that makes them more likely to become addicted to something, in ways which become increasingly hard to control. That something can be smoking, drugs, alcohol, gambling, painkillers, eating, religion, or many other options. In other words, there are certain people who are very likely to become addicts of *some* sort. They can also move from one to another, from painkillers to alcohol or from smoking to sugar for instance.

In parts of the world where alcohol is largely banned, there are very high rates of smoking and/or gambling behaviour – even if gambling is banned as well. Addiction re-wires the reward systems of the brain, giving greater mental rewards for the addictive substance or behaviour compared to things such as work, family, or even life itself.

Once someone is addicted then what the rest of us would consider rational thought goes out the window. Former Manchester United superstar George Best would have known that drinking was extremely bad for him and almost certainly would lead to his death. As many people pointed out - he had so much to live for, but still could not stop himself. After a liver transplant, he was told in no uncertain terms, 'carry on drinking and you will die.' Yet this person with 'so much to live for,' carried on drinking with the sadly inevitable result. They could change his liver, but they could not change his brain.

Then there is the case of grandmother Wendy Hamriding who had her face half chewed off by her family dog. She was an alcoholic who fell down the stairs after drinking a full bottle of vodka and who did not wake for two hours. Her dog licked her face to try and wake her, then natural instincts took over and it began nibbling her bloodied face until it had eaten her right eye and the bone around her socket.

She survived and was incredibly grateful to both the dog and the incident itself because the months in hospital and the shock helped cure her drinking problem. Even with a reconstructed face, she felt lucky to be alive because without that accident she believes her drinking would have killed her.

How bad is the addiction and how hard is it to fight, if having half your face bitten off is an easier way of kicking the habit than just stopping?

Gambling is a behavioural addiction, but the reward systems in the brain are similar to substance abuse such as drugs. Also, once again, certain people are genetically more likely to do it than others. People lose their families, their houses, their jobs and almost everything else thanks to their gambling habits. Some people end up committing suicide as the only way out of their downward spiral. If they win, then they just gamble it all away. Once again, gambling can trigger the reward system in some people's brains and the need just gets greater and greater.

Professor David Nutt of Imperial College, London, is one of the world's foremost addiction experts in the area of Neuropsychopharmacology. He helped a BBC Panorama programme into the dangers of gambling.

"Gambling addiction is not a failure of will, it is a brain disorder which is preyed upon by the gambling industry," he said. "Once you have become addicted it is very hard to stop because you have changed your brain. Addiction is a brain which has changed to become trained to the results of gambling."

Nutt and his team did a test with a former gambling addict playing roulette while undergoing an MRI scan. It would strike me as the most obvious line of research, but once again this was a 'unique experiment' which had never been done before.

It showed the brain activity that took place during the gambling session and the powerful changes that occurred. Crucially, in terms of deciding policy in this area, Nutt showed that the mental high comes from the anticipation of winning, not the result or winning itself. In other words, losing can have the same effect as winning on the brain's rewards system.

Further research has compared the brain reactions of gamblers to non-gamblers when put through a similar gambling situation. 2009 research by Cambridge University showed how the brains of gamblers reacted with the same excitement to a near miss as to a win. Non-gamblers, by way of contrast, would only get excited about winning. Designers of slot machines have used this information to programme near misses into their machines to make the experience more addictive.

Addictions do not have to be bad

Why do people go on roller-coasters, or bungee jumps, or white-water rafting? All these things, and many more, are utterly pointless in their own right, but for many people, they induce the release of various pleasurable hormones, in the vernacular they give people a buzz. That too is an addiction of sorts.

Felix Baumgartner was literally the man who fell to earth - from 23 miles up towards space, travelling faster than the speed of sound. At least he would not have been able to hear himself scream. The obvious question was why he would do something with no obvious benefit, despite the attempt to dress it up as providing various types of irrelevant scientific knowledge, but which was pretty dangerous despite the safety planning. One example was that getting into a spin would have seen blood coming out of his eyeballs, while low pressure would have led to his blood literally boiling. The psychological explanation involved his ever greater pursuit of the buzz from extreme situations. In the same way that a drug addict is less stimulated by their drug as time goes on, psychologists suggest that Felix Baumgartner was no longer particularly stimulated by jumping out of a plane at 10,000 feet. He needed something bigger and bolder.

Large numbers of base jumpers, and extreme sportspeople using wingsuits, die when their dangerous pursuit goes wrong. I question why healthy, fit, young people put themselves in a position where the odds of survival are so dramatically reduced, but I think I have answered my own question. They cannot live without the risk of dying.

A missing buzz even applies to top sportspeople when they get 'mentally tired.' Effectively that means a run of top level, intense activity, so the body does not release performance-boosting hormones to the usual level. Many coaches swear that rest is almost as important as training for the very top international sports stars. In turn, upon retirement, countless sportspeople have struggled to reproduce the buzz that their sport provided, sometimes with bad consequences. They are addicted to something their ageing bodies can no longer deliver.

Understanding others

I have never smoked or taken drugs, and I can give up drinking for periods relatively easily. It is a statement of the bleeding obvious to say I have never been anorexic. I have hardly ever gambled and certainly have no great interest in it. With the benefit of hindsight, I think I did suffer depression for a while – but it was mild, and caused by a particularly manipulated set of work circumstances. A change of job banished those feelings; in hindsight I know I was lucky compared to many.

I may not have that much personal experience of traditional addictions, however, I can look at the evidence. The extreme circumstances people will endure to maintain their addiction, the things they give up as a consequence, the risks they take, mean I appreciate the strength and power of addiction. I may not feel those things in the same way, but equally I would not dream of thinking I could change those people just by telling them what to do.

Why can't people adopt a similar approach to fat people? How come we understand that there are issues involved with addiction, PTSD, anorexia or depression, but cannot understand that the balance of the brain has an impact on obesity and it can be at least as hard to control.

When I buy a family pack of jam doughnuts and eat them in the supermarket car park, my behaviour is biologically similar in many ways to the person who gambles their paycheck on a horse, drinks a bottle of vodka before lunch, looks for that latest drug, or who jumps out of a space capsule. I am doing something that I know to be potentially damaging on a conscious level, but which my body is craving.

Why over-eating is the worst addiction of all

Addiction is something which corrupts the brain's rewards system. The more we understand that, the more chance we have of avoiding any relapse. Whether it is by using different behaviours to trigger different reactions, drugs, (even recent research into electro-magnetic stimulation), we are looking for new ways to change the brain to defeat addiction.

But whichever way the science is developing, there is one key to defeating addiction in pretty much every successful model. The way we get over an addiction is to stop altogether. In terms of smoking or drugs, we may try to wean ourselves off through substitutes of some form or another, but the end goal is always to stop completely.

Alcoholics do not become social drinkers enjoying the occasional glass of wine at the weekend – if they do then they rapidly relapse. I have lost count of the number of friends who have given up smoking for a period of time, then tried one in a social environment and ended up smoking as much as before. The long-term treatment of drug addiction is not to have occasional hits instead of regular ones; gamblers are not encouraged to beat their addiction by reducing their habit.

To take Alcoholics Anonymous as the obvious example, you never stop being an alcoholic, you have just been dry for a period of time. There is a heavy religious element to Alcoholics Anonymous, which makes sense when you realise it could in itself be a replacement addiction for some people.

The way to treat every single addiction is to stop. Pure and simple. But that is not an option when it comes to eating.

We have to eat to survive; we cannot go 'cold turkey' (not the most appropriate way of putting it, but you know what I mean).

People who overeat have to give up a little bit. We have to go from a bottle of vodka a day to half-a-bottle as a way of curing our addiction. No-one else cures their addiction that way for a reason – it is the hardest way of all, some would argue well-nigh impossible.

Not only do we have to carry on eating, but we need a certain amount of all the bad things in order to be healthy. We need some fat, some sugar, etc. We are expected to be able to control the quantities our brain is demanding. These do not reduce over time; if anything, they get harder to control. We need to carry on triggering the parts of the brain that crave these foods.

So no, I would not claim over-eating is as serious as depression or various other addictions. However, I would claim the instincts are the same and the drive as strong. The chemicals released from the hypothalamus are the same, satisfying the opiate sensors in the brain is the same, but the 'cure' is even harder. The brain of an obese person, the reward systems triggered by food, will be different to a thin person – that neurological difference is a good definition of addiction.

The US Surgeon General describes addiction as a disease and similar language is used about obesity by some educated people. I understand where they are coming from. I completely agree with their analysis in terms of obesity happening to people rather than being a positive choice; however, I am not sure 'disease' is the most helpful wording. We have to do our best to defeat it, we have to find ways to improve the situation, so I am happy to leave it as an addiction rather than going further.

Anyone who thinks eating cannot be an addiction really means it is not an addiction for them, which is a very different statement.

PART 2: THE REALITY

CHAPTER 7

How Did It Come To This – The History

"Harvard's extensive research on the subject weaves a story of ancient humans who were both extraordinarily active and able to easily gain weight in times of plenty."

Alvin Powell

There was a battle in 1689, at a place called Killiecrankie in the Highlands of Scotland, between the Jacobites and Royalists. One of the losing Royalists was running away from the winning Jacobites only to find his escape blocked by a ravine and fast-running river. Facing likely death at the hands of the pursuing soldiers, he leapt across the 5.5-metre gap from one set of rocks to the other, with only three or four uneven metres of run-up.

When you measure the distance on the ground, it is hard to imagine many people being physically capable of jumping such a distance in perfect conditions. When you see "Soldier's Leap", in real life, it looks even more impossible. Just for comparison, a little over eight metres wins you an Olympic long jump medal; that's the most-talented modern athletes in the world after years of training, with a perfect run-up, landing in a sand pit, having six goes – and not wearing battle gear! However, fear lends us wings, as they say. Our soldier cleared the jump and got away because his chasers looked at the leap a bit more rationally and did not follow. It gives a new meaning to the phrase "fight or flight".

It is a positive example of why humans have developed instinctive behaviour; how the human body can achieve amazing things without engaging the brain. Fear and desperation would have flooded that soldier's body with hormones – such as adrenaline – to maximise his physical performance in that moment of need. Hesitation, in order to debate the pros and cons, would have been fatal, so the decision to go for the jump had to be purely instinctive.

If you talk to a top sportsperson about being in "The Zone" – where they can perform at their best – it is usually the most instinctive state with the least-conscious interruptions. In other words, blocking out too much thinking is often the key to top performance. Athletes act first and think afterwards. We have evolved to act and react without thought on a regular basis in order to survive. To move to the top of the evolutionary tree, as we have, we needed these super-strong survival instincts. It has been a good thing to limit that conscious oversight on so many of the body's functions including, as it happens, our desire for food.

The best description I have seen of how our minds work is to think of the brain as an onion with a central core and layers added around it. The old parts of our brain, the parts we have in common with many animals, are still there in the central area called the basal ganglia. We share some of the next layers with more advanced animals, such as monkeys. As human beings have continued to develop, our 'onion' has added more layers unique to us. Our complicated thoughts and reasoning come from those newest layers as our brain size has increased. We have parts of the brain which set us apart from other animals, but we still have parts of the brain in common with other animals.

That is why so much obesity research is carried out on animals such as rats. You can question the ethics, but not the scientific validity of such research. They are testing parts of the brain, hormones, and hormonal reactions, which we share.

Primitive urges and instincts are still dominant; they have to be. We still need to mate, have children, and prolong the human race, so we have hormonally-driven urges to do all that. We then need to look after and develop our children thanks to maternal and paternal urges. In particular, the lengths a mother will go to in protecting her children are legendary. When the hormonal balance goes wrong, then we have issues such as post-natal depression.

We need an immune system to cope with illness. In the days before anaesthetics, people coped with extraordinary pain and these things would happen naturally with no conscious influence. They all happened for millions of years before our brains developed their outer layers and we reached our current levels of analytical ability.

Our prehistoric selves needed to keep warm, so that involved inventing fire and killing animals for fur. We needed the skill and strength to be able to kill those animals; the bigger, the better.

And we needed to eat a balanced diet to function most effectively. So that meant we needed the brain chemicals such as Leptin, Ghrelin, and Neuropeptide Y as part of our evolutionary development (of course, we have this in common with other mammals). Roughly speaking, they are the primary chemicals in your brain that make you want to eat, but also – crucially – decide *what* you want to eat and *when* to stop.

We needed to put in very particular fuels to keep the body going – even though some of those fuels could only be obtained from dangerous sources. Filling up the stomach was not enough. Otherwise, we could have eaten tree bark and leaves. Only the fuels which provided the energy the body needed would do; only certain types of food would trigger the satisfaction centres of the brain – and we needed to do all that instinctively.

As Deborah Cohen and Thomas Farley of the RAND Corporation, Santa Monica, (a global think tank for research and development) wrote in Preventing Chronic Disease in 2007, "The continued growth of the obesity epidemic at a time when obesity is highly stigmatizing should make us question the assumption that, given the right information and motivation, people can successfully reduce their food intake over the long-term. An alternative view is that eating is an automatic behavior over which the environment has more control than do individuals. Automatic behaviors are those that occur without awareness, are initiated without intention, tend to continue without control, and operate efficiently or with little effort.

"The concept that eating is an automatic behavior is supported by studies that demonstrate the impact of the environmental context and food presentation on eating. … A revised view of eating as an automatic behavior, as opposed to one that humans can self-regulate, has profound implications for our response to the obesity epidemic, suggesting that the focus should be less on nutrition education and more on shaping the food environment."[29]

Our subconscious desire to eat – our hunger pangs – needed to be so strong that they made us go out and confront life-threatening danger. If our prehistoric Risk Assessment Forms had recommended eating grass for safety reasons, then things would have turned out very differently. There is a reason cows do not rule the planet.

Survival of the fattest

At one Fat Class, a member made this comment when asked about controlling cravings, "I might not know much, but I know we are not animals." That is a sign of the social pressure fat people are subjected to, the strength of the 'willpower' message, and the constant battering of ignorance. Even some of *us* believe it, or pretend we do.

As a human race, there is one thing that is without doubt. We ARE animals. It is important to understand that while we are all different, there are some behaviours and instincts we share with each other, and large parts of the animal kingdom.

University of Kansas research published by The Royal Society[30] has shown that part of evolution over the last five million years seems to reward animal species with low metabolic rates – in other words, less activity. Those more active, with higher metabolisms, are more likely to become extinct.

Bruce Lieberman, Professor of ecology and evolutionary biology who is also a co-author for the study said, "Instead of 'survival of the fittest,' maybe a better metaphor for the history of life is 'survival of the laziest' or at least 'survival of the sluggish'."

We may be able to make some sets of decisions at a mental and conscious level, estimated at just 5-10%, but the human body has a strong set of instincts – like any animal. These have kept the species alive and allowed us to develop into iPad users. Some of them also make us fat.

The irony is that our increasing brain size is to blame for obesity. A larger brain needs lots of energy to function, much more than the smaller brains of other animals. That is why our bodies have been set up to store more energy – in other words, make us fatter. A fully fit human body will carry around 15% body fat and, of course, many of us are capable of carrying far more body fat than that. A Chimpanzee, by comparison, will carry 4-5% body fat.

Dan Lieberman, chair of Harvard's Human Evolutionary Biology Department, argues that being fat is an essential part of being human, "Mothers need … to produce milk even if they didn't eat that day. Human reproduction required us to have energy on board. The importance of fat for survival has long been paramount in humans. We evolved to crave foods we can convert into fat easily."

So, millions of years ago, we developed three key urges, triggered by stomach hormones and controlled in the primitive part of the brain. The first, influenced by our Ghrelin and Insulin-like Peptide 5, generated appetite and hunger that made us want to eat. The second, influenced by Peptide YY and Leptin, made us feel full when we had enough, while the third meant Insulin and Oestrogen dictated the efficiency of our body tissue in storing fat. That is a deliberate simplification of a complicated process; there are a few more hormones with long names floating around, literally, and even scientists do not fully understand the role of every one. One thing we do know for certain is that the whole process works through the Hypothalamus at the core of the brain. There are two sets of nerve cells there that make us feel either hungry or full and, obviously, their balance is key.

The more we chased and stored food, the better our chances of survival. For much of our history, Darwin's survival of the fittest literally meant the survival of potentially the fattest.

Our bodies and brains needed various proteins and vitamins, some from plants and some from meat, in order to grow, procreate, and look after our young. Once we found a way of cooking meat, that opened up another area of development and growth of the human brain because of the enzymes that were released. Once we found a way of farming grain, that too opened up new areas of brain and social development. Once we found ways of keeping warm, we were able to expand over more of the planet.

There is some irony to the fact that the analytical capabilities that allow us to become vegetarian or vegan were caused by brain growth that resulted in part from eating cooked meat.

The irregularity of food meant the body developed ways of storing energy in times of plenty, to be able to use those reserves in harder times. It is a part of tissue biology known as adipose tissue deposits.

Some did this better than others. For example, Jonathan Wells revealed in a paper to the International Journal of Epidemiology the case of the Pima Indians, who are Native Americans from Arizona. They were used to a desert lifestyle with short bursts of plenty followed by long periods of hardship. The result was a need to store fat as efficiently as possible during the good times to prepare for the lean times. When they became exposed to a Western lifestyle and the consistent availability of food (in other words, non-stop good times!) they developed particularly high obesity rates because their bodies were so efficient at storing the fat.

It is thought to be a similar story for the indigenous Aborigine population in Australia, whose obesity rates are at the joint highest level alongside the poorest sections of society. Again, they are historically a hunter-gatherer population used to feast or famine and have a genetic make-up to match.

These peoples are not unique; over history, the evolutionary process has rewarded those who are good at storing fat for the bad times. Some of the greatest numbers facing the obesity crisis also combine a genealogical background from areas of contrasting winters and summers, along with modern exposure to plenty of year-round food. People in places such as Northern Europe and Northern America.

Of course, as the philosopher Thomas Hobbes put it, the original state of human life before society was not a good one. "In such condition, there is . . . continual fear, and danger of violent death; and the life of man, solitary, poor, nasty, brutish, and short."

There were all sorts of causes of death in primitive times as very few lived beyond the age of 40, but high cholesterol did not figure particularly prominently. There are no reports on cancer-causing carcinogens scratched into the cave paintings! As a race, we did not need to worry about storing up long-term health problems until the last few centuries – and especially the last few decades.

Once upon a time, nature was self-regulating – if any hunting caveman started getting fat then his success rate in gathering food would fall off, the first diet perhaps and the most natural one of all. As Kelly Brownell, director of the Yale Centre for Eating and Weight Disorders, and Katherine Horgan Ph.D. put it in The Food Fight, "You are an exquisitely efficient calorie conservation machine. Your genes match nicely with a scarce food supply, but not with modern living conditions."

Our inner Jolly Green Giant did not need to limit these urges until the last 40 to 50 years; previously, we would be long gone before any potential problems could emerge. We did not need any genetic control mechanism to limit sugar intake and fat storage. In fact, the opposite worked best.

Bearing in mind that our self-regulation worked pretty well for thousands and arguably millions of years, the big question is – what went wrong?

CHAPTER 8

How Did It Come To This
– Modern Society

**"The food industry profits from providing poor quality foods
with poor nutritional value that people eat a lot of."**
Dr. Mark Hyman

Our relatively recent ability to control food supply led to another stage
in our development as a species and helped to cement our dominant
position on the planet. We have gone from lean cavemen eating raw
meat, to chubby consumers of microwave ready-meals.

That is progress.

One of the interesting things about the worldwide obesity crisis is the
way it has spread. Some countries have been hit earlier than others; some
to a greater degree than others. Either we think willpower and lifestyle
choice can be blown on the wind, or we can trace the trends which cause
global obesity.

There are some clues in terms of wealth, farming, and the food industry;
it is interesting to see that where obesity rates have slackened off, there
are correlations with slowdowns for particular sections of the food
industry.

By 1980, many advanced parts of the world already had an obesity issue;
more than 10% of people had a BMI above 30 in the US, UK, Middle
East, South Africa, Australia, Russia, and China, to name the main ones.
Rates have risen further in all those countries, but BMI has risen fastest,
since then, in Latin America, Africa, and Asia. The biggest rates of
change have been in China where obesity has increased almost eight
times, and – more surprisingly – Mali in Africa where the rate has gone
up more than 15 times. Latin America has also seen general obesity rates
rocket, with some of the highest rates of female obesity in the world.

Brazilian Professor of Nutrition and Public Health, Carlos Monteiro, of
the University of Sao Paolo, links this to industrial food processing,
which he says is now one of the "main shaping forces of the global food
system." He shows how ultra-processed food products – fast food,
packaged food, pre-prepared food – have less protein, less dietary fibre,
more free sugar, more total, saturated and trans fats, more sodium, and

more calories. To fulfil basic levels of nutrition, we take in far greater numbers of calories.

During the period 1997-2009, when obesity rates in the developing world grew faster than the developed world, sales of packaged food, soft drinks, processed food, snack bars, alcohol and tobacco in low- and middle-income countries all outstripped equivalent sales in high-income countries. Sales of rice, beans, meat, and milk all dropped in Brazil between 1996 and 2009, while bread, cookies, soft drinks, sweets, sausages and ready meals all went up. Ready meals went up the most. Obesity in Brazilian adults went up 5% between 2006 and 2012. It is estimated that Brazilian obesity percentages will catch up with the US in the mid-2020s.

A graph of how much a country uses ultra-processed foods is remarkably similar to a graph showing obesity rates. For example, Monteiro points out that Mexico, Chile, Canada, and the UK all had obesity rates of 25-30% when ultra-processed foods formed 50-60% of the diet of those countries. In countries where processed food was around 20-25% of the national diet – such as Brazil and Columbia at that time – there were obesity rates of around 15%.

The Food and Agriculture Organisation of the United Nations reported that in a 25-year period from the 1960s, the amount of food energy available per person per day went up by 450 calories in developed countries, and 600 calories per person per day in developing countries. Those levels of extra energy have been calculated to cause weight gain of roughly a pound a week.

The UN also reported a 'nutrition transition' across the board to a diet resembling that of developed nations, with an increase in sugars, plant oils, and complex carbohydrates as a significant factor among the changes.

Barry Popkin of the University of North Carolina put it simply. "Over the past several decades a dramatic shift in stages of the way the entire globe eats, drinks and moves have clashed with our biology to create major shifts in body composition."

Of course, ultimately, we decide what to put in our mouths, but it would seem mad to disregard these trends – the amount of food available, the type of food available, the aspirational example set by developed countries, and the marketing which affects an individual's decisions. The fact that available food energy has increased in every single country worldwide would also help to explain one of the stranger statistics – that obesity has increased in every single country and culture with *no exceptions*, even in countries we still associate with poverty and starvation.

Popkin is one of many who talks about the major mismatches between our biology and modern society. He elaborates, "It is useful to understand how vastly diets have changed across the low- and medium-income world to converge on what we often term the 'Western diet.' This is broadly defined by high intake of refined carbohydrates, added sugars, fats, and animal-source foods. Diets rich in legumes [beans, lentils, and the like], other vegetables, and coarse grains are disappearing in all regions and countries. Some major global developments in technology have been behind this shift."

He earmarks the increased use of particular foodstuffs. Vegetable oil(s) intake increased between threefold and sixfold, depending on the country, between 1985 and 2010, with people over the age of two in China consuming an average of 300 calories per day in vegetable oil.

Popkin points out that 75% of food and drinks bought in the US contain 'caloric sweeteners.' In particular, the amount of sugar from drinks has gone up dramatically over the period of obesity growth. "In 1977–78, two-thirds of added sugar in the US diet came from food, but today (in 2012) two-thirds comes from beverages. However, this may be an underestimate, as the USDA added-sugar estimate excludes fruit juice concentrate, a source of sugar that has seen major increases in consumption in the last decade and is now found in over 10 percent of US foods."

There is also an increase in foods sourced from animals; for example, meat and eggs, which can be good in terms of nutrition and bad in terms of some fats. Also combined with the increase in processed foods, we have seen a decrease in vegetables and coarse grains which started in the US during the 1980s and then spread to Asia and the rest of the Americas – once again mirroring worldwide rates of obesity.

Those statistics are shadowed by the increasingly global activities of the world's biggest food companies. Growth for the world's Top Ten food companies has slowed in the wealthiest countries, so many of their advances in recent years have come through expansion in developing countries. Products which were originally developed for the US market have been increasingly sold worldwide. As one tiny example of that trend, Domino's Pizza opened 1,281 new stores in 2016, but more than 1,100 of them were outside the US. Nestlé issued a press release in 2008 boasting of a 25% increase in sales to lower-income consumers in the developing world to 6 billion Swiss Francs, while adding ominously, "The overall market for such products in Asia, Africa, and Latin America is estimated at over 80 billion Swiss Francs."

A New York Times investigation, in 2017, reported a study from market research firm Euromonitor which showed a 25% growth in the sale of packaged foods worldwide in 2011-2016, compared to a 10% increase in the United States. Over that period, the rate of increase for obesity in the US has been slower as well. Soft drinks sales have doubled in Latin America since 2000 and overtaken those of North America. Fast food sales have gone up 30% worldwide, and 21.5% in the US, whilst fast food sales in Argentina, for instance, went up two and a half times.

The response of the food industry has been straight out of the tobacco industry playbook – to the extent that former tobacco industry executives have been consulted on food industry policy. Amazingly, in hindsight, the food industry was brought into government discussions by many countries as a central part of their policy-making in fighting obesity – especially during the 1990s. Having consulted the turkeys on whether they wanted to vote for Christmas, they declined.

Instead, the response of the food industry has been threefold. Firstly, they have put the blame firmly at the door of individuals' lifestyle choices and willpower. Sean Westcott, head of food research and development at Nestlé, blamed the natural tendency for people to overeat. He said to The New York Times that Nestlé strived to educate consumers about proper portion size and market foods that balance "pleasure and nutrition." At the same time, they marketed a chocolate biscuit in Brazil with a name that translates as 'Non-Stop' (Sem Parar) which hardly reinforces the education about smaller portion sizes.

Secondly, the food industry has contributed to political causes on all sides, and formed or guided lobby groups. It just so happens these moves have helped to block trends, laws, and taxes to encourage healthier eating. Once again, the main focus of blocking these moves involves trying to deflect attention towards individual responsibility in general, and often exercise in particular.

When the citizens of Berkeley, home of the University of California main campus, wanted to apply a soda tax in 2014 (one cent for every ounce), the American Beverage Society spent $2.4million opposing the plan – that's $30 for every eligible voter. The vote was still passed in that affluent area and subsequently drink sales fell by almost 10% over the following two years. No wonder the food industry was worried.

In another move straight out of the tobacco playbook, the food industry commissioned a significant proportion of the scientific research. Favourable reports were released, awkward findings locked in a draw – and this has been going on for a long time. A University of California, San Francisco, study released in 2017[31] showed the extent of this behaviour. They revealed for the first time 'Project 259' – set up in 1965, led in the UK by Dr. WFR Pover at the University of Birmingham, funded by the Sugar Research Foundation, and aimed at disproving a link between sugar and heart disease. When the research led to a link between sugar (sucrose) intake and cancer, particularly bladder cancer, the plug was pulled and the research never saw the light of day. Study co-author Stanton Glanz of UCSF said, "Had [Project 259] actually been completed and published, it would have advanced the general scientific discussion about the sugar/heart disease link. They prevented that from happening. It helped to derail this issue for quite a long time."

The same UCSF researchers also revealed, in 2017, that Harvard scientists had been paid in the 1960s to push the blame for heart disease away from sugars and towards saturated fats.

In 2015, The New York Times revealed the depth of the involvement of Coca-Cola in funding a new "science-based" solution which conveniently relies more on exercise than calorie control. "The beverage giant has teamed up with influential scientists who are advancing this message in medical journals, at conferences, and through social media. To help the scientists get the word out, Coke has provided financial and logistical support to a new nonprofit organization called the Global Energy Balance Network, which promotes the argument that weight-conscious Americans are overly fixated on how much they eat and drink while not paying enough attention to exercise," wrote Anahad O'Connor. Scientists involved in GEBN told the New York Times that Coca-Cola had no control over the work they did.

In 2011, industry group the National Confectioners Association supported research which conveniently showed, in their words, "Children and adolescents who eat candy tend to weigh less than their non-consuming counterparts." The Louisiana State University study, published in Food and Nutrition Research, held back from recommending candy as anything other than an occasional treat though. In 2016, Associated Press revealed one of the co-authors had written an email describing the paper as "thin and clearly padded."

Thirdly, the big food companies have invested heavily in the diet industry. Weight Watchers was bought by Heinz in 1978, who still provide some of their packaged food after a further change in ownership (US TV star and businesswoman Oprah Winfrey bought 10% of shares in 2015), the diet drink Slimfast went to Unilever in 2000, Nestle bought up diet meals company Jenny Craig in 2006. All the big food companies still sell the bad stuff, but put supposedly healthier products beside them – partly so they can win both ways and partly so they can once again point the finger back at individual choice and education. Sales of supposedly healthier packaged foods have also increased, so it's win/win.

While the food industry will argue they are the good guys and gals – reducing calories in some countries, being part of the diet industry, and promoting some healthy brands – there is a limit to what they can achieve in the real world without upsetting shareholders. Even if sales of foods which are marketed as being better for you have doubled, they still accounted for only 7% of food and drink sales in 2016.

The Economist magazine reported how PepsiCo chief Indra Nooy set out to sell healthier products in 2006. "In 2010 PepsiCo declined to advertise its sugary drinks during America's Super Bowl, launching a marketing campaign for social causes instead. Shareholders began to revolt. They wanted PepsiCo to give its full support to money-making products, healthy or not," explained the magazine.

In 2013, PepsiCo sponsored the whole half-time show at the Super Bowl, arguing Pepsi drinks and snacks were an essential part of watching the sport on TV.

The New York Times quoted Coca-Cola International president Ahmet Bozer telling investors in 2014, "There's 600 million teenagers who have not had a Coke in the last week. So the opportunity for that is huge."

Food processing

Refined sugar is a relatively recent addition to the diet of the masses. The relevance of the 'refined' part of that statement is that it makes the sugar easier to absorb, harder to use naturally (therefore more likely to be stored as fat), and also more addictive – a triple whammy. For a long period of our evolution, refined sugar was not available at all; then, for the last few centuries, it was only available for the rich few. In the last century, it has become more widely available, spreading most in cheaper diets in the last 50 years. It is one of the ironies nowadays that obesity is a problem which hits the poor hardest, where once only the rich were fat. There's equality for you.

There is a persuasive argument that the obesity crisis is not caused by the amount we eat, but *what* we eat. Much of modern food is unnatural compared to our historical diet. Some foods are more likely to be turned into body fat than others – for instance, milk chocolate versus more natural dark chocolate, or high fructose corn sugars versus honey, to take just two examples. In both cases, the body copes better with the latter.

There are many who argue about the dangers of high fructose corn syrup, because it is such an unnatural sugar for our bodies to digest. The cheap by-product is used in animal feed to fatten animals up for market; it seems it has the same effect on humans.

High Fructose Corn syrup (HFC) came from increased corn production in the US in the 1970s, initially under President Nixon as a response to the increasing cost of food which threatened his re-election hopes in 1971. Farmers were persuaded to grow corn on an industrial scale which resulted in a surplus and a desire to find more uses for the produce. In the mid-1970s, ways were found of mass producing a sweet syrup from the surplus corn. HFC was incredibly cheap, made food tastier, and was soon used as an ingredient in almost any processed food from pizza to coleslaw. Not only did it make things taste nice and sweet, it also dramatically improved the preservation of those foods. Use of HFC in the USA between 1970 and 2007 increased ninefold.

There is real biology behind the theory that HFC is spectacularly bad for us. The cell structure of HFC and refined sugar is harder for the body to use up as energy, making it more likely to be stored as fat, compared to natural sugars such as glucose or honey.[32]

We know rats fed on HFC or mono-sodium glutamate (MSG) will put on more weight than rats fed the equivalent amount of calories in healthier food. We also know rats' bodies react differently to HFC compared to equivalent amounts of more natural sugars, again putting on more weight.

It is easy to say we are different to animals such as rats, but there are also enough physiological similarities between us to take note of the research. Both HFC and MSG are frequent ingredients in processed, pre-prepared food. In the UK alone, the ready meals business is now worth £3billion. In order to make them last long enough, and taste good enough to buy again, those pre-packaged dinners (including 'healthy options' meals) include all sorts of additives. Even bags of salad have chlorine and acids to keep them looking fresh.

In his book, Child Health Guide: Holistic Paediatrics for Parents, Dr. Randall Neustaedter writes, "High Fructose Corn Syrup is twenty times sweeter than sucrose (more natural sugar), cheaper to make and convenient for food manufacturers because it retains moisture and blends well with other ingredients. The free fructose in corn syrup interferes with the heart's use of minerals, depletes the ability of white blood cells to defend against infections, and raises cholesterol and triglyceride levels. Fructose inhibits the hormones that make us feel full (insulin and leptin), and it triggers the hormone that makes us feel hungry (ghrelin). Children do much better on diets free of corn syrup. Most commercial, sweet, processed food products contain high fructose corn syrup. These products include candy, soda, energy bars, sweetened yoghurt, energy drinks, and baked desserts."

Dr. Richard Johnson, in The Sugar Fix, links the American obesity epidemic to increased use of fructose. "Americans consume 30% more fructose today than in 1970. Our rising consumption of this sugar began at roughly the same time that obesity rates in the United States were climbing sharply. ... These corresponding trends are intimately linked."

He puts forward a persuasive case, both in terms of the statistics and the scientific logic. However, it cannot be the entire story. HFC use has dropped in the US while obesity rates continue to climb, albeit more slowly. The same statistic applies to carbohydrates, incidentally; another popular target in the obesity debate.

We also know from research in China that increased doses of MSG in food will lead to increased body weight in apparently healthy adults. This is particularly relevant because MSG is perceived as a major component of pre-prepared Chinese food worldwide; we also know it is a commonly used part of animal feed.

What we feed our farm animals is inevitably going to end up in our bodies. If we use growth hormones on the animals, then we are changing nature's balance and ultimately our own body balance. How the animal is fed makes a difference. We know cows fed on grass will produce milk with more Omega 3 than those given cattle feed, for example.

Not how many, but how

Sugar is a blanket term for a lot of sweet products. We need some sugar in our diets, but not all sugars are created equal. Unrefined sugar is not as bad as refined sugar, but it seems liquid sugar is worse again. This helps to explain the strong correlation between soda drinks in particular and obesity, though concentrated fruit juice drinks are almost as bad.

Of course, these drinks have huge quantities of sugar, famously a can of Coke has around 10 spoonfuls of sugar, similar to most sodas, sports drinks, and fruit juices. However, it is not just about the amount of sugar; it is also about how liquid sugar fails to trigger the brain response that enough is enough.

Purdue University, Indiana, research in 2000 and 2009, showed how bodies responded less to liquid sugar intake than solid sugar intake in terms of suppressing appetite – for example drinking apple juice compared to eating an apple.[33] Eating had a longer effect on suppressing appetite than drinking, meaning the calories in a drink are largely extra to normal intake. People who ate an apple, or even an equivalent number of calories in jelly beans, would eat less, later, than those who had a sugary drink. Basically, our Inner Jolly Green Giants include solid sugars in their daily dietary demands, but ignore liquid sugar.

Also, liquid sugar has been found to affect insulin sensitivity and increase the risk of Type 2 diabetes in several studies such as the 2009 research by the Department of Molecular Biosciences, Davis, California[34].

Liver disease[35] and heart disease[36] have been added to the list of risks – with drinks sweetened by High Fructose Corn even worse than other sugars.[37]

These results all match the studies looking into the effect of soda drinks consumption and obesity rates, with the adverse effects of liquid sugars being greater for women than men. A 2006 report by researchers from the Harvard School of Public Health and the German Institute of Human Nutrition[38] looked at 30 relevant reports over a 39-year period.

They concluded, "Findings support a positive association between soda consumption and weight gain, obesity, or both. Sugar-sweetened beverages, particularly soda, provide little nutritional benefit and increase weight gain and probably the risk of diabetes, fractures, and dental caries (tooth decay or cavities). Consumption of sugar-sweetened beverages such as soda and fruit drinks should be discouraged, and efforts to promote the consumption of other beverages such as water, low-fat milk, and small quantities of fruit juice should be made a priority."

In 2013, the American Journal of Public Health printed a report by scientists from Stanford, London, and Cambridge Universities along with a scientist at the World Health Organisation.[39] They studied international soda drink sales and compared them to obesity rates. The two have a pretty close alignment all the way from low soda drink sales/low obesity, through to countries with high soda drink sales and high levels of obesity.

While it is undoubtedly a factor, it is not as simple as saying soda consumption equals obesity rates. If you look at graphs comparing the increase in soda drinks, general sugar, and even carbohydrate intake and obesity in the US, then we see the two lines rising almost identically from 1980 to 2000; after that, soda drink, sugar, and carbohydrate levels drop slightly while obesity continues to increase.

One explanation for that recent divergence could be the increased use of sweeteners as a replacement, which are almost as bad as the original sugars. A 2018 study by the Medical College of Wisconsin and Marquette University is the largest ever held to track biochemical changes in the body after consuming sugar or sugar substitutes. "Despite the addition of these non-caloric artificial sweeteners to our everyday diets, there has still been a drastic rise in obesity and diabetes," said lead researcher Brian Hoffmann. "In our studies, both sugar and artificial

87

sweeteners seem to exhibit negative effects linked to obesity and diabetes, albeit through very different mechanisms from each other.

"We observed that in moderation, your body has the machinery to handle sugar; it is when the system is overloaded over a long period of time that this machinery breaks down. We also observed that replacing these sugars with non-caloric artificial sweeteners leads to negative changes in fat and energy metabolism."

The researchers couldn't decide which was worse, sugar or artificial sweeteners, but the fact the debate was happening in the first place is instructive.

The sweeteners are less natural and harder to digest. The way and the reasons they end up stored as fat – affecting our insulin resistance and threatening diabetes – are different to natural sugars, but the end result is worryingly similar. As nutritionist Brooke Alpert, the author of The Sugar Detox, points out, "Artificial sweeteners trigger insulin, which sends your body into fat storage mode and leads to weight gain."

Sugar substitutes act as a trigger of the hunger hormone ghrelin, because the body expects sugar but does not get it, so rather than being part of a solution to obesity they simply add to the problem. An American study of 23,000 adults[40] showed people who were overweight or obese drank more sugar-free drinks than people of normal weight. The overweight group ate more, and one theory is that this was at least partly to compensate for the cravings triggered by the sugar-free drinks.

Famous Five a Day

The UK Government's advice is for us to eat "Five a Day", meaning five bits of fruit or vegetables in a balanced diet. There is analysis that we actually need to eat anything up to 70(!) a Day because modern farming and consumerism means that fruit and vegetables have less of the nutritional goodness they used to. Especially in the UK, where we are more focused on the uniform appearance of fruit and vegetables than their mineral and vitamin content. To go back to the bagged salads, they are estimated to have four times less health-boosting antioxidants by the time we open them compared to when they were first bagged.

That could be one explanation as to why we now eat so much more to satisfy our bodies; we need to eat more food to get the same nutrition. There are increasing cases where people are both overweight AND under-nourished – an amazing combination due to the low nutritional quality of some modern, fattening food.

Certainly, one of the key points for top sports nutritionists – the people feeding our elite sportsmen and women – is the organic quality of the food rather than different basic ingredients to what the rest of us might eat. What they eat is high quality produce and better balanced to provide the range of nutritional needs. Food is organic in the original sense of the word, and without additives. Production methods are more important than a stamp or a label of certification.

The USA is the country with the best food consumption record-keeping over the last 40 years, and the statistics make interesting reading for those who believe tackling obesity is as simple as reinforcing the Five-a-Day message.

For a start, the figures show the amount of food energy per person in the US stayed stable through the 1970s when obesity rates started their modern rise. However, from 1980 it increased steadily by around 20% per person, with carbohydrates and fat increasing by a similar amount.

Interestingly, there are also signs of the health messages getting through – though that may also be a part of the problem. The US Department of Agriculture reported, in 2009, that red meat consumption was down, while chicken more than doubled; fresh fruit and vegetables both went up by a quarter; refined sugar was down by around 40% while diet soft drinks increased by two thirds. We have looked at the problems with diet drinks, but that is not the only bad news in the figures. Some 'health messages' getting through were equally damaging, resulting in butter and whole milk use going down substantially (I'll return to why that is a bad thing). All these figures were very much in line with the health messages being pushed, for better or worse.

There were also some clear explanations as to why obesity rates were increasing in the figures: cheese tripling, further HFC increases, alcohol going up, and overall soft drink consumption also substantially up.

However, it is not just what we consume which offers a clue to the problems. There is also an issue about how we get hold of our food.

In this period, the convenience food industry was the strongest growing part of the food economy. The number of restaurants, cafes, and snack bars doubled, whilst sales of prepared meals at grocery stores quadrupled over the 1980s and 1990s.

Barry Popkin talks about the increase in convenience store chains, particularly in the developing world, and their growing influence on how people spend their money on food. Improvements in distribution chains and the shelf-life of food have allowed them to squeeze out many local producers, process more food, and transport it further. "For example, in Latin America, supermarkets' share of all retail food sales increased from 15 percent in 1990 to 60 percent by 2000. In comparison, supermarkets accounted for 80 percent of retail food sales in the United States in 2000. This process is also occurring at varying rates in Asia,

Eastern Europe, the Middle East, and all urban areas of Africa," he wrote.

'Globalisation' is an obvious way for a trend to spread globally – good or bad. The more we get our food from an environment where we are exposed to sophisticated marketing, the more we are likely to make bad choices.

Deborah Cohen of the Department of Health, RAND Corporation, Santa Monica, looked into how marketing affects the way people respond sub-consciously. "The increases in food marketing and advertising create food cues that artificially stimulate people to feel hungry. Many internal mechanisms favor neurophysiologic responses to food cues that result in overconsumption.

"External cues, such as food abundance, food variety and food novelty, cause people to override internal signals of satiety. People's natural response to the environmental cues are colored by framing, and judgments are flawed and biased depending on how information is presented. People lack insight into how the food environment affects them, and subsequently are unable to change the factors that are responsible for excessive energy consumption."

In other words, when we are pushed by availability and marketing towards a greater variety of food choices then we consume more. A combination of neuro-imaging of the brain and behavioural experiments show how we react subconsciously to food marketing and availability. 65% of all buying decisions were made in the store with 50% not planned in advance.

Put simply, if we go to buy carrots at a shop which only sells carrots, then we will return with just carrots. If we buy carrots at a shop which also sells candy bars, then there is a much higher chance we will buy carrots and candy bars. The likelihood of that is enhanced further by a promotion or other marketing tools (using very similar tactics to a magician 'forcing' our choices as it happens). There is an extraordinary level of statistical research into buying habits, both individually through store cards and generally through overall trends, along with the neurological research into the behaviour of the supermarket customers. It shows the supermarkets how to tempt our subconscious decision-making. Put simply, they are getting better at selling us things whether we want (or need) them or not.

By tracking our subconscious decisions and comparing them, supermarkets may even know if someone is pregnant before they do themselves!

It is also worth pointing out that candy bars – and processed food in general – can make far more profit than carrots, or 'purer foods' overall.

The ingredients of a packaged meal can be as little as 5-10% of the final cost. That means there can be an awful lot of people taking a slice of the multi-processed cake.

We are influenced much more than we imagine. For example, a British study[41] showed that restaurant diners will spend 10% more if there is classical music in the background, compared to no music or pop music. In particular, they will spend the extra on appetisers and coffees, the theory being that classical music creates an upmarket mood. It is very unlikely those customers realise their choices of starters are affected by the music in the background.

Most supermarkets have the fresh fruit and vegetables close to the front of the store as one of the first areas where we go to pick up our groceries. That is because their research – and practical data – shows we are more likely to buy 'treats' after buying some of the 'good stuff' first. Once we have vegetables in our trolley, we are more likely to give in to the marketing in the crisps aisle, for instance.

It all hinges on us not realising how easily we can be manipulated; in us thinking we have complete conscious control over our decisions – or should do. The Willpower Myth allows this manipulation to spread, along with obesity. It's another example of how it is society which has become obesogenic, as much (or even more so) than individuals.

CHAPTER 9

The Blame Game

"Fat is usually the first insult a girl throws at another girl when she wants to hurt her. I mean, is 'fat' really the worst thing a human being can be? Is 'fat' worse than 'vindictive', 'jealous', 'shallow', 'vain', 'boring' or 'cruel'? Not to me."

JK Rowling

Kara Florish describes herself as being less than national average weight, certainly not obese, so the last thing she expected to encounter on a London Underground train was fat-shaming. However, a middle-aged, white man handed her a card as he left the train which shocked her and many who read her subsequent Facebook picture and post in December 2015.

"Overweight Haters Ltd," read the Fat Card, "It's really not glandular, it's your gluttony...

"Our organisation hates and resents fat people. We object to the enormous amount of food resources you consume while half the world starves.

"We disapprove of your wasting NHS money to treat your selfish greed. And we do not understand why you fail to grasp that by eating less you will be better off, slimmer, happy and find a partner who is not a perverted chubby-lover, or even find a partner at all.

"We also object that the beatiful (sic) pig is used as an insult. You are not a pig. You are a fat, ugly human."

Another overweight woman handed such a card, just for having the audacity to travel on a London Underground train, was left in floods of tears as the young perpetrator skipped off, not facing the result of his actions. Did she really make a 'lifestyle choice' to be left crying on a train?

There would be two reasons for crying in that position. Of course it was an act of upsetting cruelty, but – probably, more importantly – it would remind you of the years of dieting, discomfort, and unpleasantness that had not worked as well as hoped.

The cards were reported to British Transport Police, and they also prompted a social media backlash. Although they were on a small scale, these Fat Cards are an extreme example of the core belief shared by so many in the obesity debate. Most people – 75% in the biggest American survey – share the basic view that obesity is the fault of fat people's greed. They also believe – thanks to the weight of negative headlines about the price of obesity-related treatment (and despite the longer-term evidence to the contrary) – that *our* obesity is costing *them* money.

That drives them to tell fat people what they consider 'home truths'. It is all part of the perception that fat people just can't be bothered to put the effort in to be thin. As a result, "We need to be told!"

One part of the Fat Card explained, "We do not understand why you fail to grasp that by eating less you will be better off, slimmer, happy". This could be the core theme of thousands of diet books, DVD's, articles, TV and radio programmes or social media advice.

Weight for it

In a four-year study[42] of just under 3,000 British adults, those who reported day-to-day "weight discrimination" gained more weight than those who did not. The report also suggested that weight discrimination even spread to many doctors, who underplayed the role of genetics in obesity and treated patients disrespectfully – leading to less than helpful interactions and outcomes.

"Most people who are overweight are aware of it already and don't need it pointed out to them," said Dr. Sarah Jackson, of University College London, one of the authors of the report. "Telling them they are fat isn't going to help – it is just going to make them feel worse. There are lots of different causes of obesity, yet a lot of blame just seems to be on individuals and a lack of willpower. Raising awareness of some of the factors involved might make it easier not to blame people."

Dr. Brenda Major and others at the University of California have also looked at the effect of 'stigma' on overweight people. They found that criticism typically made overweight people eat more calories, not less. Non-overweight people were not affected by negative coverage.

In the Journal of Experimental Psychology in 2014[43], Major and her colleagues wrote, "America's war on obesity has intensified stigmatization of overweight and obese individuals. Exposure to weight-stigmatizing news articles caused self-perceived overweight women, but not women who did not perceive themselves as overweight, to consume more calories and feel less capable of controlling their eating than exposure to non-stigmatizing articles. Findings suggest that social messages targeted at combatting obesity may have paradoxical and undesired effects."

As Dr Arya Sharma, a professor of obesity at the University of Alberta, Canada, put it, "A widespread misconception, even amongst well-meaning folks, is that spreading the word about the dangers of obesity and using overt or even just subtle social pressure to "nudge" people to improve their health behaviours for their own good, is a reasonable approach to solving the obesity problem.

"That such "shame and blame" tactics generally misfire should be no surprise to the many individuals actually affected by this condition.

"It is certainly bad enough to have to suffer the negative emotional and physical consequences of excess weight – being blamed for the problem and being constantly reminded just how bad it is without being offered any reasonably effective solution can only make the whole situation even worse."[44]

I didn't know they made XXXXL Hair Shirts

Hair shirts are part of our weird and horrible history, a punishment for someone who supposedly deserves a penance for their sins. Wearing one was a sign of repentance and/or atonement. It was extremely irritating and unpleasant by design.

There is archaeological evidence that wearing something to irritate the skin pre-dates written history. It was part of Judaism in Biblical times and has been carried down through Christianity, particularly the history of the Catholic Church. However, the principle of unpleasant repentance has some form in all religions.

Hair Shirts were usually made of goat hair, or they could be girdles if you wanted to make things even more irritating. They were painful, itchy and sore, meant to be a constant reminder of the sin. Sackcloth could do the same thing with less bother. Hence the large role that sackcloth plays in religious traditions. Deluxe models would include wire or twigs for extra discomfort!

Many of the major characters of religious history demonstrated their true devotion in such a way. For instance, Archbishop of Canterbury Thomas Becket was wearing one when he was killed in 1170 for putting his religion and church ahead of his King, Henry II.

The modern day equivalent is being fat.

Or at least that's how it feels.

The central premise of the hair shirt, or its equivalents, is that you have sinned and you deserve to suffer. That is also the starting point for the treatment of many fat people. We deserve something unpleasant to make up for breakfasting on doughnuts.

Many of us take our punishment on a daily basis in terms of the diets we choose. We are made to feel guilty about being fat because it is perceived to be our choice and something we can easily address. There are plenty who believe in the 'cruel to be kind' approach to fat people. Many of us believe it ourselves; we deserve to suffer.

I will call this the Hair Shirt Treatment; we lost the right to a good life when we chose to be fat. But, this is a problem in a few ways, two in particular.

Firstly, as we have already discovered, feeling that we have sinned, feeling under attack, feeling we are in the wrong, triggers all the emotional hormones that eating nice stuff can satisfy. In other words, being made to feel we have sinned makes us sin even more.

Secondly, in the search for solutions to the obesity crisis there is a huge bias towards the Hair Shirt Treatment of fat people rather than more pleasant – and crucially more effective – programmes. The approach is one of telling fat people "This is what you must do" not one of "Let's find out what you *can* do." It means telling us to do unpleasant things because we deserve it, rather than reasonable things which will help. We are not compelled to do these things, but there is huge social pressure – both directly, in terms of the advice given, and indirectly, in terms of the praise/criticism for doing/not doing the following. So here is the advice – and what it really means:

You should eat more salads. (They will not satisfy you, but you lost that right when you chose to be fat.)

You should go to a gym more. (Of course, it may be uncomfortable and embarrassing, but you need to show you're not lazy.)

If you wear clothes that show you are fat, then you are slovenly, even though clothes large enough to go over everything just make you look even bigger. (You lost the right to wear clothes that fit when you chose to be fat.)

Every time you food-shop, you have to spend at least five minutes in the 'healthy eating' aisle. (You will have to buy food that will not fill you up, that will have almost as many calories as nicer and more fulfilling stuff. You lost the right to buy normal food when you chose to be fat.)

There are people who believe we deserve to pay more for seats on an aeroplane, we deserve to pay more for clothes, even that we deserve to pay more tax.

The worst fat-shaming I have ever seen was on SKY TV's Obese - A Year To Save My Life when the lady at the centre of the programme was filmed showering naked. Her fat hung down and covered her modesty, if that's a good way of putting it. What level of human dignity has been stripped away from someone that the programme-makers would film such things and she would agree to it? It meant they believed she deserved such fat-shaming – and so did she.

Those depressing mistreatments of a human being were caused by the school of thought that we can be 'shamed' into deciding not to be fat. It is a poor excuse for being inhumane, but it is all-too-common.

Milking the issue

We know fat-shaming is counter-productive, but there is another, potentially bigger, problem. Too many pieces of diet advice are based on the Hair Shirt Treatment at the expense of effective behaviour.

For example, we are regularly told we should use the low-fat versions of everything. That is often bad advice on a couple of levels. I will start my explanation with the example of milk.

Almost every article, study, diet plan, bit of advice and guidance I have seen, tells me to have skimmed milk if possible; or semi-skimmed if I cannot cope with fully skimmed milk. Every 'diet' recipe includes semi-skimmed milk at best and increasingly soy milk, or some equivalent, because it has less saturated fat.

Skimmed milk is pretty unpleasant on cornflakes, but it has less than 1% fat so it must be good for me, surely? They even do a version that is lower fat than skimmed milk. It makes your cornflakes taste revolting.

But here's the thing – skimmed milk has almost the same calories as full-fat milk. Full fat milk is only 4% fat in the first place, so the name is not remotely accurate. I will call it normal milk instead. If we put skimmed milk in our tea or coffee, for instance, we are likely to put more in to get the taste we are looking for. That means we will put in more calories than using a smaller amount of normal milk for the same results. By using skimmed milk, there is a high probability we will be taking in more calories than if we use normal milk.

Amazingly, though, it gets worse. I will go into the health debate much more fully in the next chapter, but the fat in milk is very natural and is one of the key building blocks for a healthy life. It has been shown to make 'fat people's diseases' such as Type 2 Diabetes less likely. "People who had the most dairy fat in their diet had about a 50 percent lower risk of diabetes compared with people who consumed the least dairy fat," reported Dariush Mozaffarian, Dean of the Friedman School of

Nutrition Science and Policy at Tufts University in Boston, Massachusetts, who is an author on a 2016 study.[45]

Also, by drinking skimmed milk we may be missing out on fat-soluble nutrients like vitamins A and E. Skimmed milk is literally just milk with most of the good stuff taken out, but almost all the calories left in.

So by using normal milk, we are likely to take in fewer calories with greater health benefits.

Some people prefer the taste of semi-skimmed milk, it is less rich and you do get used to it. However, if you want watered down milk and fewer calories, then try watering down the milk literally – water does not have any calories at all.

Low fat, big problem

It is a similar story with butter. Remember sales falling 12% in the US in line with the 'health messages' that butter is bad for you, and lower fat margarines are good? Up until the 1980s, most margarines contained up to 20% trans-fats, which are strongly linked to heart disease. They have also been linked to increased obesity, as they are harder for the body to use naturally.

Methods of making margarine have been changed as a result. Most are now made in a way which means they contain little or no trans-fats, though vegetable oil-based margarines are likely to contain some. These 'hydrogenated' fats are produced when vegetable oil is hardened. They improve the shelf life of processed foods, and are used in biscuits, pies, and cakes. Also pretty much anything that has been heated by frying, so any takeaways are likely to be high in trans-fats.

However, you will not see trans-fats on the food labels. You need to look for hydrogenated fats or hydrogenated vegetable oils, but that is only a rough guide as not all of these will convert into trans-fats during the production process.

But the main point is the complete misconception that butter is bad for you just because it contains natural fats, compared to margarine with manufactured fats. The biggest and most reliable research on the matter shows that butter usage has no noticeable effect either way on heart disease or cholesterol levels. In fact, Type 2 Diabetes was the only area where researchers found a difference in using butter. They found butter users 4% LESS likely to develop the illness.

You can argue whether other foodstuffs, such as olive oil, are even better than butter but the 'health messages' which have driven a 12% drop in butter use – despite its lack of any negative effect on health and its marginal benefit for helping avoid diabetes – shows how mad prejudice can be.

The same applies to many low-fat foods, which we are encouraged to use so strongly. Take natural yoghurt as one example. Full-fat natural yoghurt, according to plenty of evidence, is a healthy food that helps lower rates for illnesses such as Type 2 diabetes. It has the equivalent of one teaspoon of sugar as a natural by-product. Zero fat natural yoghurt has around six spoonfuls of sugar and/or sweeteners to compensate for the lack of fat. Without the sugar or the fat, it would taste horrible and hardly anyone would touch it. Yet sugar is more clearly a cause of the problems than fat, both in terms of weight and health, so we are being pushed towards the less healthy food by some alleged experts.

A report by the Division of Public Health Sciences in Seattle[46] put together the results of 16 studies on the links between high-fat dairy and obesity along with heart health. They concluded, "The observational evidence does not support the hypothesis that dairy fat or high-fat dairy foods contribute to obesity or cardiometabolic risk, and suggests that high-fat dairy consumption within typical dietary patterns is inversely associated with obesity risk."

So they seem to have come to the reluctant conclusion that high-fat dairy products are linked to a *lower* risk of obesity, while stressing the importance of how the food is produced as a key factor in the healthiness of what we eat and drink.

Likewise, a 2013 study published in the Archives of Disease in Childhood, a British Medical Journal publication,[47] showed that children are also less likely to be obese if they have normal milk and dairy products.

"For a long time we've had this notion that saturated fat is always bad for you," said Mark DeBoer, a paediatrician at the University of Virginia and one of the authors. "It appears that children who have a higher intake of whole milk or 2 percent milk gain less weight over time compared with kids who consume skim or non-fat dairy products."

Chocolate can be good for you

You can hear the horror. I can almost feel the coffee being spluttered into my face. But there is growing evidence that this statement is true – chocolate can be good for you.

For example, there is a Tel Aviv University study which shows that chocolate cake or cookies for breakfast can help weight loss. It's based on a study of almost 200 obese, non-diabetic adults put on a sustained diet for almost eight months. They were split into two groups, one given a 300-calorie low carb breakfast every day, the other a 600-calorie breakfast including chocolate cake.

The length of time was important because for the first four or so months the weight loss between the two groups was similar. But then the bodies of the low carb group rebelled and they started putting weight back on. The chocolate cake group carried on losing weight and at the end of the eight months had lost an average of almost three stone more. That's a remarkable result.

Professor Daniela Jakubowicz of Tel Aviv University, who conducted the study[48], said, "The participants in the low carbohydrate diet group had less satisfaction, and felt that they were not full, but the group that consumed a bigger breakfast, including dessert, experienced few if any cravings for these foods later in the day."

Seems simple. More importantly, it seems attainable. It's one of the very, very few pieces of research which addresses the hormonal changes around eating. Maybe doughnuts for breakfast would be a good thing, after all.

All fat people know how cravings build up through the day, leading to bingeing – like a dam bursting – in late afternoon or late at night. It may be that day; it may come after a few days. It's not enjoyable; it leaves you feeling guilty, miserable, and awful. Having something calorific for breakfast gives your metabolism all day to use the energy while reducing your ghrelin levels for the rest of the day compared to the low-carb breakfast. In layman's terms, that means putting your Inner Jolly Green Giant to sleep for a while.

This study makes complete sense in so many ways. It was published in 2011, so why is it not official weight loss policy in loads of countries by now? Or at least mentioned in passing? Why do we not have celebrities pushing their favourite chocolate cake breakfasts on the front covers of magazines?

You can't help feeling the answer to that is simple. Chocolate cake for breakfast would be too nice. It doesn't matter if it might work, fat people don't deserve it. They deserve the Hair Shirt Treatment instead.

But here's an interesting question. Why is chocolate one of the body's go-to comforts? Is it because it is actually good for us?

Researchers in Finland[49] found chocolate reduced the risk of stroke by an amazing 17% in the group of men they tested. It reduced bad cholesterol and increased good cholesterol. It has loads of antioxidants, which take out bad free radicals. It is high in minerals and has also been shown to have a small effect in reducing blood pressure. It may help prevent heart disease and the flavonoids in cocoa beans improve the functions of the brain in old age.

These benefits apply primarily to dark chocolate, or well-made chocolate. They do not particularly apply to the sugar-enhanced commercial milk or white chocolate brands. We are back to the debate about the way in which historically healthy foods are made unhealthy modern foods by multi-national companies.

Once again, though, there is no-one pushing the benefits of a daily slice of dark chocolate. It's still chocolate – and fat people don't deserve chocolate.

BMI – Blooming Mathematical Idiocy

The biggest rise in obesity literally happened overnight. To be strictly accurate, between the 2nd and 3rd of June, 1997. For on the 3rd of June, the World Health Organisation (WHO) changed the definition of being overweight from a Body Mass Index of 27 to a BMI of 25. As humans have got progressively bigger through history, not including obesity, a change in that direction makes no sense. Millions of people became overweight overnight, and the change meant the WHO was able to label obesity an 'epidemic.' In terms of tracing the origin of the Blame Game, that's a pretty good place to start.

It raises two questions – how reliable is BMI and why draw the lines where we do?

BMI works out the optimum weight for each height, below 18.5 is underweight, 18.5 to 25 is supposedly a healthy weight, 25-30 is overweight and above that is obese. To describe it as a blunt instrument is an understatement; it makes no allowance for body shape, muscle mass, or any other difference between body shapes.

Most sporty people would be classed as overweight or obese. The vast majority of international rugby players have a BMI in the overweight or obese category, while they are all ridiculously fit with incredibly low body-fat levels. Athletes in power sports such as weightlifting will be categorised as obese. Most top-level sports stars requiring any element of force, such as field athletes – basketball's LeBron James, even – are categorised as overweight. Usain Bolt, the fastest man in history, was borderline overweight with a BMI of 24.9 at his athletic peak.

The definition of 'obese' has shifted towards the BMI description, but traditionally the word involved being 'grossly fat.' To describe a load of people who are not the least bit fat as 'obese' seems plain daft and should undermine the whole BMI definition.

Jacques Peretti explains in the book The Deals that Made the World, how this change from 27 back to 25 was based on pre-war statistics gathered by the Metropolitan Life insurance company in New York. At that time, the statistics were used as a way to justify putting up insurance rates for people in the 25-27 BMI bracket. US author Joel Guerin analysed the approach of Met Life statistician Louis Dublin and concluded, "It wasn't based on any kind of scientific evidence at all. Dublin essentially looked at his data and just arbitrarily decided that he would take the desirable weight for people who were aged 25 and apply it to everyone."

Professor Judith Stern, vice president of the American Obesity Association, told Peretti, "There are certain risks associated with being obese … but in the 25-to-27 area it's low-risk. When you get over 27 the risk becomes higher. So why would you take a whole category and make this category related to risk when it isn't?"

The logic behind the decision gets even weirder when researchers in Copenhagen[50] showed the BMI level associated with the least risk of dying had gone up steadily, in a survey covering more than 100,000 people over 37 years. In fact, for the group studied between 2003 and 2013, the 'healthiest' BMI had risen to 27.

Given that the arbitrary move away from 27 and down to 25 in the 1990's was itself based on questionable methods relating to 25-year-olds and pre-war data on death rates, it is amazing it has not been adjusted back up. However, Met Life started the process of making money out of a lower rate for obesity and they have been far from alone in the decades since.

Lowering the BMI numbers and increasing the number of overweight people in the world also increases the focus on the issue and the blame on those people. This change in BMI categories simply opens up the Blame Game even more. There has been controversy over so-called Fat Letters. These are sent out by schools and designed to warn parents about overweight primary school children in England.

The letters are based on taking a BMI measurement of the schoolchildren and then determining if they are overweight. We have seen that BMI should be a highly nuanced measurement; but not for the busy-bodies who designed the Fat Letter scheme, where pupils in England are weighed in their first and last years at Primary School.

For example, there was the case of Sarah and Paul Hurry whose five-year-old son Max was healthy, slender and active - weighing 3st 2lb (19.95kg) and measuring 3ft 6in (1.07m). Despite his healthy lifestyle, they received two Fat Letters. "I felt like I was being accused of being a bad parent," Mr. Hurry told Sky News. "I felt frustrated and a little angry."

No wonder. There's a definite stigma in getting such a letter. In the end, even the Royal Society for Public Health called for "reform of, or an end to, the letters."

"Our research finds that only one-fifth of parents find the 'fat letter' useful," chief executive Shirley Cramer said.

"We believe that the letter should be seen as the beginning of a dialogue with parents, not simply flagging whether their child is obese.

"It is unacceptable that one in five children leave primary school classed as obese and we must all pull together to reverse this worrying trend."

I am not underplaying the importance of childhood obesity in any way; of course, it is a growing problem and I believe it should be the front line of the battle against obesity at all levels. However, letters such as the above are a misguided way of doing it; they are either offensive or pointless. They are consistent with the Hair Shirt Treatment that fat people, or in this case parents of possibly fat people, deserve official ridicule. They are about public shaming, not help.

Spurious correlations

There is a very funny website which has now been turned into an entertaining book, Spurious Correlations by Tyler Vigen, where he finds lots of trends which have no obvious connection. For instance, there is a curious, or spurious, statistical correlation between the number of films Nicholas Cage does in a year and the number of people in the US who drown in swimming pools. When he makes four films the number goes above 100, but drops to around 90 in the years he only makes one film.

The divorce rate in Maine matches the amount of margarine people eat, the marriage rate in Kentucky each year matches the number of people who drown falling out of a boat. My favourite two are the correlation between Japanese car sales in America and the number of suicides through car crashes, and the age of Miss America against the number of murders by steam, hot vapours and hot objects (until a remarkable departure from the similar trends in 2009!). Whenever a 24-year-old has been voted Miss America, there have been at least seven murders by steam, hot vapour and hot objects. When the age of Miss America is 20 or younger, those drop to two or three – until 2009.

No-one would argue we need to cap the number of films Nicholas Cage can make each year, or impose a lower age limit on the Miss America contest, for safety reasons on the basis of these figures.

While these are entertaining, it seems to be pretty much the level of science for so much of the obesity debate. There are lots of fat people, Type 2 Diabetes has gone up. There are lots of fat people, certain cancers have gone up. There are lots of fat people, heart disease has gone up. There are lots of fat people living longer, dementia rates have gone up.

Why? Some fat people have these conditions, some don't. It seems very unlikely that being fat is the complete – or sometimes even partial – explanation. It seems much more likely that a combination of genetics and lifestyle choices contribute substantially to the answers. It needs further research, greater understanding, but if all you are looking for is an XXXXL Hair Shirt, then there is no need to go the extra mile.

Many of us have bodies which are genetically designed to crave food and store fat. We live in a society which is increasingly disastrous for those bodies – and trying to shame fat people only increases the problems.

The blame game is not fair or accurate - and it makes obesity levels even worse.

CHAPTER 10

In Fatness and in Health

"Healthy emotions come in all sizes. Healthy minds come in all sizes. And healthy bodies come in all sizes."

Cheri K. Erdman

Ultimately, most of us are killed by our parents.

I don't mean we have loads of elderly axe murderers roaming the streets, but that most people are killed by their genetics. Whatever kills your parents has a pretty good chance of killing you. If they died of heart attacks, then you are likely to die of a heart attack. If they died of cancer, then there's a good chance so will you. If they died young because of a genetic condition then, unfortunately, you are at a higher risk of suffering the same.

Just as genetics play a significant role in whether or not we will be overweight, so genetics play an even greater role in *when* and *how* we are likely to die.

It is time to focus on the lies, damned lies, and statistics that underlie the debate over obesity and health. Why is this so important? The biggest stick used to beat fat people is the perceived cost of our selfish gluttony. The phone-ins, the articles, the official reports – they all moan about how much obesity is costing. To paraphrase the view, it's all very well for us to stuff our faces with doughnuts for breakfast, but not when it costs everyone else in extra taxes or insurance premiums to pay for our treatment.

In order to ease the pressure on fat people, in order to help us move towards proper and achievable solutions, that is one of the biggest myths that needs to be busted.

As one small example of how we are focusing on the wrong things, I was told about the unfortunate death from a heart attack of someone in his early fifties. "Of course he was very big, not just tall, but also big," it was explained. His size was described in great detail, eventually being followed by, "- and his father died of a heart attack at the same age!" Genetics were clearly a factor, but we have been brainwashed into thinking being overweight is the key to everything.

It is a myth that has been perpetuated by some of the most important people on the planet. When he was on his way to becoming President of the USA, Barack Obama said, "Just to emphasize how important prevention and cost savings can be in the Medicare system, it's estimated if we went back to the obesity rates that existed in 1980, that would save the Medicare system a trillion dollars."

One of the reasons for the controversy over his subsequent healthcare policy, nicknamed 'Obamacare,' was the idea that people had to pay for the carelessness of others. It's a view summed up by Health Administrator Austin Schanzenbach writing in the Foundation for Economic Education in 2016 under the headline, "Now you pay for your Neighbor's Weight Problem: Thanks, Obamacare. Health-conscious people have to subsidize healthcare costs for people that make poor choices."

Head of the UK's National Health Service Simon Stephens said, "Cutting down on junk food diets, couch potato lifestyles, cigarettes and booze could make Britain one of the healthiest places to live in the world, while saving taxpayers billions on future NHS costs."

In 2015 Professor Sally Davies, the UK's chief medical officer, said there should be a national risk plan in place for obesity, just as there is for terrorism. Professor Nick Finer from University College London's Institute of Cardiovascular Science went further and argued obesity is now, "The most pressing health issue for the nation. Estimates of the economic costs of obesity suggest they will bankrupt the NHS. Elevating the problem of obesity to a national risk could help to address the current 'laissez-faire' attitude to this huge, angry, growing health catastrophe."

In any obesity debate, it does not take long for the costs of medical treatment to come up. Estimates in the UK vary between £4-6 billion each year, for example. In the USA, the treatment of ill health caused by being overweight will rise to $555 billion by 2025, according to an estimate by the World Obesity Federation. They estimate the worldwide cost will reach $1.2 trillion in that time. If you compare the current figures with the substantially higher predictions for the future there may be some exaggeration in there, which suits those with an axe to grind, but it all fuels the scare-mongering.

On the face of it, the numbers and the headlines look very worrying and persuasive. It is a simple fact that obese people are more likely to have certain medical complications than thinner people of an equivalent age – and treatment costs money. Surely that's Game, Set, and Match to the anti-obesity brigade? Doughnuts, nil; small bowl of sugar-free granola, one.

Well, I'll come onto the facts and figures which show this to be the wrong approach, but first it always seemed an argument with a whole host of holes to me. It seemed the aim of all these comments was to lambast fat people rather than provide any rational analysis.

The big figures are based on a lot of individual cases and each individual is far more complicated. On a personal note, I injured my knee playing rugby when I was 18. There was no keyhole surgery in those days, so I carried on for more than 30 years with loose cartilage floating around, wearing away the rest of the joint.

Eventually, I had an operation. I was overweight. I am sure I would go down in the figures of obese people costing the NHS, but it could equally have been categorized as a sports injury that took 30 years to catch up with me. I met a lot of people in hospital who needed knee operations; many attributed the origins of the problem to sport or manual work. A small percentage of the hundreds I encountered at various stages were overweight.

When you look at the rising numbers of these operations, increasing effectiveness is also a factor. People who would once have had to put up with the pain can now get a long-term surgical solution. Some of those people may also be overweight.

Mistaken myths

The definitive study into the cost of treating obese people compared to other groups was carried out in 2009 by a team led by Pieter van Baal of the Dutch National Institute for Public Health and independently funded by the Dutch Government.[51] Their conclusions flew in the face of the popular view.

They studied three distinct groups in Holland: obese people, smokers, and a healthy living group who were non-smokers with a BMI in the 'healthiest' range between 18.5 and 25. Up until the age of 56, the health costs for the obese group were the greatest – largely because of diabetes and muscular-skeletal problems (dodgy joints in layman's terms). After the age of 56, the smokers took over as the most expensive section, with lung cancer among the obvious health problems in that group.

However, the crucial statistics concerned how much treatment costed over individuals' full lifetimes. Then we see the costs of treating the healthiest group becoming the largest overall as they get older. "Because of differences in life expectancy, however, lifetime health expenditure was highest among healthy-living people and lowest for smokers. Obese individuals held an intermediate position," explained the report.

"Although effective obesity prevention leads to a decrease in costs of obesity-related diseases, this decrease is offset by cost increases due to diseases unrelated to obesity in life-years gained. Obesity prevention may be an important and cost-effective way of improving public health, but it is not a cure for increasing health expenditures."

It is vital to underline that the most expensive issues were age-related and not linked with obesity. On average, the healthy living group lived to 84 and their treatment cost $417,000 per person, the obese group lived to 80 and cost $371,000 each. The smokers were the bargain basement, living to 77 and costing around $326,000. So the healthier we are at younger ages, the more likely we are to cost a fortune in our extended old age.

"This throws a bucket of cold water onto the idea that obesity is going to cost trillions of dollars," Patrick Basham, a professor of health politics at Johns Hopkins University in Baltimore, told The New York Times.

As one of Britain's leading think tanks, The Adam Smith Institute, put it, "Having us all slim, svelte, sober and pure of lung into our 90s would cost the NHS very much more money than the current level of topers, smokers and lardbuckets does."

Age Concern

Then there is the fat-bashing myth that this generation will be the first to have a lower average life expectancy than the one before.

People have been living longer and longer, but the argument put forward by the likes of Michelle Obama and British chef and food campaigner Jamie Oliver is that obesity means today's children will not live as long as their parents.

It's a nice little soundbite, seems an attractive idea to the fat-bashers, and somehow means fat people are even to blame for reversing human progress!

It is almost certainly untrue.

Current increasing obesity rates are not negatively affecting the life expectancy figures, which continue to go up. During the period of the obesity crisis sweeping the world from 1990 to 2013, for example, life expectancy went up an average of 6.4 years.

There are a variety of reasons why it is likely our children will continue to live longer than their parents, primarily that we are getting better at treating most diseases. That includes heart attacks and strokes, which are associated with higher numbers of obese people (even though strokes are, in fact, a greater problem for the healthy-living group who live longer). Funnily enough, obese people who have heart treatment are more robust than thin people who have heart treatment, so are likely to live longer after the first incident.

Also, fewer people are smoking, so that will have a greater impact on raising the life expectancy figures than obesity will bring them down. Remember smokers die earlier, on average, than overweight people.

"If you take Britain as an example, the probability of dying from the sorts of things caused by being overweight has gone down by a factor of four," Sir Richard Peto, Professor of Medical Statistics at Oxford University, told the BBC.

Just as we are getting better at keeping people alive in general, so we are getting better at keeping fat people alive.

The diabetes debate

I went through a gym test recently. Within three or four minutes I was asked if I was diabetic. I was there to build up the muscle around a dodgy knee, to get fitter and stronger; there was no reason to think of other health issues. But I'm fat, so the question was asked. I'm not diabetic, by the way. Then I was asked if I'm on heart medication. I'm not.

I went to see a nurse about another unrelated issue. As I started to explain, I was interrupted and asked if I was there because of blood pressure problems. I wasn't. She took my blood pressure anyway. It was normal.

We need to get back a sense of proportion. There are so many negative headlines and reports about how unhealthy fat people are, so too many assume that to be fat is to have health issues.

So, let's look at the realities. Type 2 diabetes is the illness most associated with obesity, so that is a good place to start. Diabetes is when insulin production or effectiveness in the body is impaired. Insulin helps our bodies use up sugar productively to provide energy. If insulin is not there at all (Type 1 diabetes) or reduced (Type 2 diabetes) then there is too much sugar in our blood, and that has a gradual and negative effect on most of our internal organs – if not quite from head to toe then at least from eyes to feet. In a best-case scenario it can be easily reversed, in a worst-case scenario it will kill.

Almost one in three obese people is reckoned to have diabetes; around 85-90% of those with diabetes have a BMI above 25. It seems pretty conclusive.

The headline figure, as reported in British medical journal The Lancet in 2016[52] was that diabetes had roughly quadrupled worldwide in the previous 36 years, from 108 million to 422 million. It affects more men than women, both in terms of the overall numbers and the percentage increase. It increased faster in low-and-middle income countries than in high-income countries, which is interesting because obesity grew more in high-income countries over the same period.[53]

Diabetes is plainly a significant issue, but is the recent increase down to weight or lifestyle? It is an important distinction. The former is very hard to change over a period of years; the latter should be easier to address. Certainly, it is *not* the simplistic case that being fat automatically means having diabetes,

In fact, it might be that the most effective way of reducing diabetes is to forget about obesity altogether, because focussing on that is plainly not reducing the numbers. Let's say Habit X – something like refined sugar or low-fat dairy – contributes to diabetes and fat people are also more likely to do Habit X. That means more fat people are likely to have diabetes. We know telling them to lose weight is not effective over a longer period of time; however, telling them to avoid Habit X should be easy to achieve. It may also help with weight loss as well.

Let's avoid the prejudice and look a little more dispassionately at the figures for diabetes. Given that it can affect people right across the BMI spectrum, should we be looking for lifestyle factors to explain why it is skewed towards the higher end?

People often assume the increase in diabetes is all because of obesity. However, The Lancet research team attribute more than 70% of that increase to population growth and aging – or a mixture of all three factors.

With diabetes, genetics are, once again, a key factor. A 2018 Oxford University study[54] showed the gene (KLF14) – which helps cause belly fat, externally and around internal organs such as the liver – will also affect your body's ability to control insulin, blood sugar, and cholesterol. It could be as simple as those with a genetic propensity to be overweight are also more vulnerable to diabetes.

Lack of sleep is linked to diabetes.[55] It has an impact on insulin resistance as the body tries to compensate for energy lost through that lack of sleep. Tiredness can also encourage snacking and overeating for the same reason, which is a bit of a double whammy.

2018 research by the Washington University School of Medicine in St Louis[56] argued that air pollution plays a major role in causing Type 2 diabetes, responsible for as many as one-in-seven cases in the 2016 period they were studying. The global research estimated that pollution contributed to 3.2 million of the new cases of diabetes that year by reducing the bodies' insulin production.

There are various ways the symptoms of diabetes have been put into almost immediate reverse, before any weight loss. Bariatric surgery sees blood sugar levels returning to normal long before weight loss could be a factor. Reducing calorie intake to 800 a day also sees more rapid effects than the scale of weight loss. Low-level physical activity reduces the chances of diabetes, as does drinking coffee. It seems clear the weight itself was never the sole problem.

On the flip side of that debate, increasing soda and fruit juice consumption levels have mirrored the increase in diabetes; various studies have linked red meat (though some argue this has been greatly exaggerated) and, especially, processed meats with the chances of having diabetes.

These are possible explanations for part of Habit X; why being fat is not simple cause and effect.

Sugar and Swedes

The independent Swedish Council on Health Technology Assessment came up with a study in 2013 which threw out many of the assumptions concerning diabetes.

The headlines were that low-fat diets were not necessarily the way forward, and that saturated fat was a positive influence. The recommendation was that we should eat butter, full-fat cream, and streaky bacon. There is a far greater understanding that some previously demonised cholesterol can be a good thing; indeed, there is a significant difference between good and bad cholesterol.

The one thing that comes across clearly in the Swedish study is that a low-fat diet seems to be a significant factor in causing Type 2 diabetes, and that there can be good calories and bad calories. "When all recent scientific studies are lined up, the result is indisputable: our deep-seated fear of fat is completely unfounded. You don't get fat from fatty foods, just as you don't get atherosclerosis from calcium or turn green from green vegetables," Professor Fredrik Nyström, one of the study authors, told the Corren newspaper.

"There are many mantras we have been taught to accept as truths:

- "Calories are calories, no matter where they come from."
- "It's all about the balance between calories in and calories out."
- "People are fat because they don't move enough."
- "Breakfast is the most important meal of the day."

"Of course these are not true.

"This kind of nonsense has people with weight problems feeling bad about themselves. As if it were all about their inferior character. For many people, a greater intake of fat means that you'll feel satiated, stay so longer, and have less of a need to eat every five minutes. On the other hand, you won't feel satiated after drinking a Coke, or after eating almost fat-free, low-fat fruit yogurt loaded with sugar. Sure, exercise is great in many ways, but what really affects weight is diet."

Researchers at Gothenburg University have also shown that the rates of death among those with Type 2 diabetes have been greatly exaggerated, with huge falls in the UK and Canada where they carried out their research.[57] The rates are also at a historical low, which clearly implies that obesity may be driving up diabetes levels, but these extra fat people are also better at coping with the condition. We also know the rates of more serious or costly diabetes complications are rising more slowly in proportion. Certainly, there are plenty who keep the worst effects of diabetes at bay through a changed emphasis on their diet. For some people, mild Type 2 diabetes can actually be a good thing because it moves them towards a healthier lifestyle to keep it under control.

The Lund University Diabetes Center underlined the message and recommended eight portions of full-fat milk, cream, cheese, and butter to give you a lower chance of developing diabetes. The study covered 27,000 people for 14 years, 3,000 of whom developed diabetes. They also found that regularly eating meat increased the potential for diabetes, with the biggest impact coming from low-fat meat rather than fatty meat, in findings presented to the European Association for the Study of Diabetes in 2014.

A Prospective Urban Rural Epidemiological (PURE) study[58] published in The Lancet in 2017, based on results from 135,000 in 21 countries, both rich and poor, also suggested a moderate intake of dairy fats may help to protect against heart disease and stroke.

So, already the picture is more complicated. After all, if there has been one group of people who have cut out or drastically reduced butter, full-fat milk, full-fat cheese, and cream, it is overweight people. It is something actually manageable that we have been badgered and badgered to do as part of almost every mainstream diet.

Why is all this important? The number of overweight people with Type 2 diabetes is plainly too high, and there is a worrying trend in younger age groups, so why am I trying to argue against that link? Surely, we need to keep our foot on the neck of fat people, so to speak, for their own good?

I keep looking at pictures of stick-thin experts saying all you have to do is lose weight to reduce the chance of getting diabetes. It is easy for them to say, but all the figures show losing weight over a period of time is somewhere between difficult and impossible. If it does turn out to be about diet adjustments, moderate lifestyle changes and/or other factors rather than weight alone, then that is easier to target effectively. If we are missing the point about the causes, then we may also be missing the point about the cure.

Root costs

When people talk about the costs of obesity, the costs of treating the effects of Type 2 diabetes are a large part of that debate. You can have Type 2 diabetes and cost the NHS nothing at all because the best treatment is nutritional change, or very little because some of the diabetes drugs are relatively cheap. The big costs come with complications such as amputation. That area is responsible for around 80% of the costs of diabetes, but life expectancy is years rather than decades after that, so there is a long-term saving – to be brutally honest about it.

Newcastle University researchers[59] concluded that Type 2 diabetes is caused by the fat in the liver and pancreas which inhibits the production and spread of insulin. The report says:

"It has been possible to work out the basic mechanisms which lead to type 2 diabetes. Too much fat within liver and pancreas prevents normal insulin action and prevents normal insulin secretion. Both defects are reversible by substantial weight loss.

"A crucial point is that individuals have different levels of tolerance of fat within liver and pancreas. Only when a person has more fat than they can cope with does type 2 diabetes develop. In other words, once a person crosses their personal fat threshold, type 2 diabetes develops. Once they successfully lose weight and go below their personal fat threshold, diabetes will disappear.

"Some people can tolerate a BMI of 40 or more without getting diabetes. Others cannot tolerate a BMI of 22 without diabetes appearing, as their bodies are set to function normally at a BMI of, say 19. This is especially so in people of South Asian ethnicity."

The fact the same levels of fat can bring such different results means there is a huge hole in the argument about obesity and diabetes. So what causes the personal fat threshold? We know from the Swedish research that the threshold changes according to what people eat.

There has been massive coverage of the increase in Type 2 diabetes at a younger age as the obesity crisis grows. Losing weight is likely to help prevent Type 2 diabetes. Going from 24 stone to 20 stone, for example, makes you less susceptible than someone who goes from 16 stone to 20 stone. The process matters more than the result, or the lifestyle more than the weight.

There is one more confusing piece of evidence, from the BBC Horizon programme with twin doctors and medical researchers Chris and Xand van Tulleken. Chris went on a no sugar, lots-of-fat diet and his blood sugar levels went up. Xand went on a lots of sugar/no fat diet and his body simply produced extra insulin to cope. In other words, no sugar brought the threat of too much sugar in the blood closer; lots of sugar moved the threat further away. It was just a TV programme, but carried out by two research scientists in an area where twins are used for the most reliable studies. It's not proof, but it adds to the questions about what really does, or does not, cause diabetes.

While it is not this simple in every case, there are plenty of examples where the most effective treatment of diabetes is straightforward healthy living. One example is the Whittington family, made famous in a TV documentary and book, Saving Dad. There is a lot more to it, but the short version is that Dad lived on takeaways, worked long hours as a security guard, and was around 20 stone. He had diabetes and was close to needing his leg amputated, when his two sons stepped in. Although they were fit young men (one ran half-marathons) they were also on the pre-diabetic spectrum. That shows there was probably a strong genetic element in their story which can be underplayed.

Dad was not naturally a big man – he seems to have been a Lifestyle Fattie – so they made the sort of changes that are comparatively easy. For a start, eating a high number of takeaways would mean a lot of processed foods with High Fructose Corn and Monosodium Glutamate. He stopped the takeaways, and they started exercising as a family group, building up to 100-mile cycling events. All his diabetic symptoms went into reverse, and he is now a normally healthy man in his 60's. It is a heart-warming story which is worth reading or watching in greater detail. It illustrates the huge importance of diet and activity/exercise in addressing Type 2 diabetes.

Giving fat people a leg to stand on

Diabetes is just one of the causes attributed to the huge spending on fat people by the NHS. The other major cost is musculoskeletal – things such as knee and hip replacements. As a result, fat people – and smokers – are facing being dropped off hospital waiting lists in places like the Vale of York and Wales. Never mind the reality that it is a dishonest way of manipulating waiting list figures to make up for inadequate management and funding, it is the fact that fat people are considered a reasonable target that prompts my concern.

In many places, there is a weight limit you have to be above to qualify for Bariatric surgery. In other words, you may be forced to put on weight to get the surgery that could help you lose weight. You could not make it up.

I have been through knee surgery. I had to lose weight because of the load-bearing capacities of the metalwork holding my re-aligned knee together, which was, of course, a good thing.

As part of that process, I attended a series of NHS classes to help with my weight reduction. They were called something formal and flattering; I called them Fat Classes. They were very informative, but not in the way that was intended. They did not do much to help me lose weight, but they did an awful lot to show why the NHS has failed so completely to come up with any practical help or solutions. The lessons reinforced the failed messages of the last 40 years; people were encouraged to show the right attitude rather than do the right thing. The sort of information in this book was glossed over in order to talk more about a weekly aqua-aerobics class.

Often, the physical musculoskeletal operations will help fat people far more than a National Health Service nutrition and diet course because they will help them to be more active. The attempt to delay operations for fat people is actually counter-productive.

As Clare Marx, president of the Royal College of Surgeons, commented after a survey showed that a third of clinical commissioning groups in England were delaying treatment for overweight people, "Blanket bans that deny or delay patients' access to surgery are wrong.

"NHS surgical treatment should be based on clinical guidance and patients should be dealt with on a case-by-case basis. In some cases, patients might need surgery in order to help them to do exercise and lose weight."

In turn, University of Delaware research shows that many people put on more weight after knee operations, which is counter-intuitive because you think people would be much more active after surgery.

"For physical therapists and surgeons, the common thinking is that after a patient's knee has been replaced, that patient will be more active," said Lynn Snyder-Mackler, Alumni Distinguished Professor of Physical Therapy at UD in 2010.

"But the practices and habits these patients developed to get around in the years prior to surgery are hard to break, and often they don't take advantage of the functional gain once they get a new knee."

So, putting off operations such as a knee or hip replacement will be counter-productive because those 'practices and habits' will be more deeply entrenched the longer they are delayed. The muscles, tendons, and ligaments around the knee will also change over time to protect the joint; surgery will be more effective if carried out before those changes are too great.

A 2014 study at the Hospital for Special Surgery in New York, followed the progress of 7,000 patients, and found that "Patients who were obese prior to joint replacement were more likely to lose weight than those who were of normal weight or overweight, but not obese."

The people with the most to gain from early surgery are the very people health trusts are looking to delay for at least 12 months. The financial problems in the NHS are clear, but making fat people a scapegoat is not the correct solution. These pieces of research show the people with the least to lose from a delay to their knee or hip operations are actually those with lower BMIs.

So, to sum up, there is a hugely over-simplistic Hair Shirt approach to the costs related to obesity. It is often portrayed as simple – fat people cost more. However, it is nowhere near as straightforward as that. The final word can go to UCLA's Traci Man in Secrets from the Eating Lab. "Variables such as exercise, weight cycling (losing and gaining weight), socio-economic status, fat distribution, and discrimination all factor into a person's overall health… I hope you're not still under the impression that you have to diet or obesity will kill you. If you exercise, eat nutritiously, avoid weight cycling, and get good quality medical care, you do not need to worry about obesity shortening your life. Especially if you shield yourself from weight stigma and the stress it causes."

CHAPTER 11

Do You Believe Me Yet?

**"Each and every one of us has unknowingly played
a part in the obesity problem."**
Indra Nooyi

There are three things I need to show you in this book, which all fly in the face of most advice:

- We need to understand the real truth behind why we are fat.
- I need to show why you should **never** go on a short-term diet again.
- We need a plan which will work for each of you.

Hopefully, we are a long way towards the first two, which in turn sets up a chance of the third.

There are plenty of 'experts' who might take a different view, many thin people may not yet be persuaded, and even some fat people may have the standard arguments so ingrained (along with guilt) that they are not wholly convinced.

However, the facts and figures go only one way – and it's not the way of the standard messages. Bluntly, the 'Eat Less, Exercise More' view that has held sway for 40 years has simply presided over the obesity crisis getting ever worse. It has been a distraction at best, damaging at worst. With every dieting course, the vast majority of articles, and TV programmes and radio interviews, all saying different versions of the same thing – the problem has escalated. That advice is either wrong or ineffective – either way, it is time to change.

Many health industry professionals, doctors, and dieticians will still disagree. So how can that be?

Well just as human nature means many of us are overweight, so human nature means the debate has not moved on. There are three main reasons:

- Cognitive Dissonance.
- We do not try to learn from failure.

- We are not as rational as we believe.

Starting with the first reason – what is Cognitive Dissonance? It's a theory first put forward by social psychologist Leon Festinger in 1957 which has a vast body of research case history backing it up. It has stood the test of time and is a mainstay of psychology textbooks.

We think we believe in something and then act accordingly. Festinger explained how it is often the other way round; our actions can affect our beliefs. What we do dictates what we think. If we have invested time and emotional effort into something, then we are likely to believe in it more – even when proved wrong. I'll give the entertaining example in a moment, but first the science-y bit.

Festinger's first experiment was very simple. People were asked to carry out a very, very boring task (such as turning pegs in a board for an hour) and then tell a third party it was a really exciting and fun thing to do. For their trouble, half of the experiment's participants were given $20 to effectively tell a lie (a lot of money in 1957) while the other half were given just $1. Afterwards, they were asked to describe the original activity in their own words.

So, surely, the people given more money would find the process of telling the lie more rewarding and be more positive, right?

Wrong, as Festinger predicted in advance. Because the $1 group were not lying in return for a reasonable reward, they persuaded themselves they were not lying at all, and the dull original activity really had been fun. The alternative was admitting they lied for next to no reason. In contrast, the $20 group admitted the original activity was boring in reviews after the event.

It was one of many examples that showed how we are less likely to admit something is wrong if we have invested time and effort into it, even when the evidence is plain. Festinger, and many others since, have shown how the actions we have taken affect the beliefs we hold.

Now the funny example from the book When Prophecy Fails. Festinger was able to infiltrate a religious group, led by a lady called Dorothy Martin (initially re-named Martha Keech in his book to protect her identity) who had also been involved in the origins of Scientology. She believed the world was going to come to an end through flooding on December 21, 1954, but true followers would be picked up from her house by a spaceship and saved.

She persuaded a group of followers to give up their jobs, leave their families, give away their money and possessions, to go to her house and wait for their cosmic rescue. December 21, 1954, came and went without a flood or rescuing spaceship, much to the group's puzzlement and dismay. Eventually, Martin claimed their devotion had been recognised with the delay of the apocalyptic event; it had not happened *because* they were ready for it – a brilliantly inventive get-out clause.

The group was ready to sign up for this explanation against the alternative of admitting they had been a bit stupid. Even odder, the group – who had been deeply secretive and private in the build-up to the 'end of the world' – were happy to do public interviews and shout from the rooftops afterwards to defend their actions.

It is the same with the diet and food industries. While obesity rates rise worldwide, they will not admit their spaceship has not come. They have to blame someone else, so they blame fat people.

They have invested too much in their personal actions, the advice they have given, belief in their own mental strength, the profits they make, to admit they may be wrong.

Which brings me onto the second point on failing to learn from failure. Festinger's theory of Cognitive Dissonance is covered in detail by Matthew Syed in his book Black Box Thinking, but the main thrust of that book is even more pertinent.

The book explains why we learn more from analysing failure than covering it up. Syed gives two over-arching examples:

- Aviation, where every crash or mistake is analysed in detail through the Black Box records, with lessons learned in as much depth as possible. There is no cover-up because a bad crash or near miss usually means airlines are better able to deal with that problem next time.
- Healthcare, where the main driver is to cover up mistakes – partly because of ego and partly to avoid insurance claims. As a result, those mistakes are more likely to be repeated, and lessons are not learned.

Obviously, there is far more detail in Black Box Thinking, but I was struck by one area Syed doesn't cover – the fact the diet industry never analyses failure.

People are hailed for going on diets, celebrated as champions when they lose all their excess weight, pictured on the front covers of magazines, before and after pictures plastered over the newspapers. Indeed, how many pictures have you seen of a newly thin person holding out their old, over-sized clothes to show how much weight they have lost?

But there is little analysis of what happens next, when more than 80% of the time the weight goes back on over the next few years. We look to learn from the short-term successes, not the long-term reality.

The Channel 4 show, Super Slimmers: Did They Really Keep the Weight Off? was a rare programme which illustrated this point perfectly. They followed six weight loss prize winners a few years on from those publicity shots with their old clothes. Five of them had put much of the weight back on in the subsequent years. The sixth remained thin – but he had originally become overweight through a lifestyle of takeaways and went on to become a personal trainer, so maybe he was not your average fat person on either count.

Jane Hall was Rosemary Conley's "Slimmer of the Year" in 2012 after losing eight stone on the programme that once rivalled Slimming World and WeightWatchers in the UK by including an exercise session in their weekly meetings. Despite Hall's clear determination, she had put much of that weight back on since. The TV show took her to meet Conley, who has made a fortune through low-fat books and weight loss programmes; her Hip and Thigh Diet book alone sold two million copies.

The return of Hall effectively confronted Conley with one long-term outcome to her methods, but her reaction was classic. Instead of recognising the limitations of a short-term approach, it re-affirmed her original methods as having worked once and being needed again. Conley has invested – and gained – a lot from her diet advice. She did not seem able to contemplate the idea that it does not work long-term, even with Hall standing in front of her. There was no new learning from studying and understanding failure.

Conley is far from alone; no-one follows up their failures. Suzanne Mendonca, a New York-based police officer who lost 90lbs on The Biggest Loser in 2005, told The New York Post, "NBC never does a reunion. Why? Because we're all fat again."

It's a theme picked up by the Museum of Failure based in Helsingborg, Sweden. Curator Samuel West explained to Business Insider, "Even the biggest, baddest, most competent companies fail. The trick is to create an organizational culture that accepts failure so that you can fail small ... rather than failing big."

So by holding out the Holy Grail of being thin, as all those blockbuster diets do, and ignoring the subsequent failures, as they also all do, we fail big – appropriately enough. We need to learn to fail small, which means accepting and understanding those failures.

System failures

Nobel prize-winning psychologist Daniel Kahneman wanted to know more about how we think. We like to think of ourselves as being like

Mr. Spock from Star Trek (in that every decision is a calmly analysed assessment of the situation and probable outcomes) when, in fact, we are much more like the emotional Captain Kirk or even the super-emotional Scotty.

New York-based Kahneman talks about two different thought processes in his book Thinking, Fast and Slow. System 1 thinking is quick, emotional and instinctive; while System 2 is slower, more fully thought out, logical and Spock-like. The two methods use different sides of the brain, separate areas which developed at different times of our evolutionary progress. We work out the answer to 2+2 on one side, 27x13 on the other, for example.

Kahneman showed that while we often *think* we are using the analytical System 2 to make decisions, we are actually using the more instinctive System 1. System 1 is faster so, by the time System 2 is clicking into gear, the decision has already been made. System 2 is largely used to justify System 1 decisions.

He gave the example of someone who is quiet and studious; someone who likes reading books. Then he asked if that person was more likely to be a librarian or a farmer? Most people gave 'librarian' as the answer to the question – the instinctive response about the quiet, studious book reader. The analytical answer was that there are 20 times the number of farmers as librarians, so there are likely to be far more quiet, book-reading farmers.

Kahneman also got people to offer any amount of money they wanted for a good bottle of champagne. The only extra requirement was that they had to pick an apparently randomly numbered ball out of a bag before doing so. A group with just high numbers in the bag offered substantially more money for the champagne than a group with just low numbered balls in the bag. A low number meant offering nothing at all up to £15 for the champagne. The people who drew a high number out of the bag offered £40-65 for the bottle. In other words, our decision-making process could be dramatically manipulated by creating an instinctive mindset thanks to the apparently random number on a ball!

Curiously many of the participants would go into detail about why they were offering the amount of money they did, although the point was very clearly that their 'rational analysis' was just a System 2 justification of their manipulated System 1 decision.

Kahneman won his Nobel Prize for economic theory, going some way towards explaining how lots of extremely clever people caused the 2008 banking crisis that brought chaos to the world's economies. His explanation of loss aversion – that we will chase losses to win them back more than we preserve winnings – is fascinating.

It also helps to explain one of the great contradictions of being overweight. If we all try hard so much of the time to lose weight, why can we rarely succeed? I think the answer lies partly in Kahneman's revelations. A desire to lose weight is System 2; the cravings to eat more are System 1. He explains why decisions we do not want are so much more powerful than those we do. His studies are aimed far above this level, but it helps to explain why we end up eating a biscuit when we know we shouldn't!

Swimming with the tide

It all comes back to what made me start this book. At that time, I knew there were plenty of people on what I'll call the 'other side' of the debate who had a deeper background in nutrition and dietary science than me. The one thing that made me think I had something worthwhile to contribute was that I knew it was not as simple for me as they made out. I am overweight, and I do not want to be. I train regularly, I try to eat well, but I am still overweight. I have felt my body fighting back, I have seen things work one day and not the next. It is not just me being weak – the figures show I am not alone.

I knew it was not as simple as an attitude of mind because I live it every minute of every day. Every day of my life I am either hungry or guilt-ridden.

I would love to be thin; I would love to be able to stick to an effective diet. I get little or no pleasure from eating; it is functional rather than desirable. It avoids a negative rather than being a positive. I knew the popular messages did not work for me, that it was more complicated, that it had more to do with the unconscious brain than a conscious decision to eat too much.

So, I felt I had a new voice worth listening to and started doing the research. I thought I would be swimming against the tide. I thought I would be arguing against the research and the scientific knowledge.

What I have discovered is that there is actually a vast amount of research which completely explains and backs up my views! I discovered there are many, many doctors and university professors – experts in their fields from the world's top universities – who have produced research that explains what I think and do.

I do not believe I am, after all, swimming against the tide of scientific opinion. What I am doing, is swimming against the tide of popular prejudice and self-serving ignorance. The more science I read, the more I find evidence which backs up my views. In fact, it became really hard to find any proper research which backs up the popular prejudices.

When I started specifically looking for studies which contrasted with my views, I found newspaper articles, blogs, self-serving arguments from the food and diet industries, plenty of short-term examples – but precious little long-term research which still stands up to scrutiny.

It has been eye-opening. Not only are all the popular messages failing, they have been scientifically debunked.

The more research I did, the more the question changed. It was not a question of 'why is there no research backing up the views of overweight people?' It became a question of 'why is all this research so largely ignored?'

As just one example, there is the 2011 Israeli research (mentioned already) that a group who had chocolate cake for breakfast lost three stone more (over eight months) than a group on a traditional calorie-controlled diet. The core message has been backed up by scientists at Maine and Syracuse Universities in 2016[60] on the benefits of dark chocolate for breakfast in helping the brain and reducing cravings. The cocoa in dark chocolate satisfies the brain's receptors. It succeeded without the sugar and fat, which is why milk and white chocolate should still be avoided. One of the key points about the Israeli research was the way the chocolate affected appetite hormone levels through the day. North Carolina neuroscientist Will Clower went further along those lines in the self-explanatory book Eat Chocolate, Lose Weight.

Why has the research not been repeated, or tried over a longer period of time? Why has no-one found a way of debunking it, showing what was wrong if they can? I have found arguments against the chocolate cake for breakfast approach from dieticians and nutritionists, none of whom mention the hormonal element which seems central to me. I found one article that knocked the eight-month study on chocolate cake for breakfast as too old and too short-term to be reliable, before pushing an egg breakfast study which had taken place over eight weeks!

So why do we continue to push people towards a diet which is shown to be three stone less effective? Why is that research never mentioned in official guidance? You can bet that if a group eating nothing but lettuce had lost three stone per person more than a group eating chocolate cake, then we would have heard plenty about that.

That was why my research took me away from the science of diet and weight loss and into the world of psychology, to try to understand why people follow their prejudices rather than the evidence. The science of obesity was becoming so clear; the real puzzle was why we stuck strongly to outdated and discredited views.

This chapter shows how people have an instinctive reaction to obesity, which they then look to justify. If they have invested time and effort in the 'Eat Less, Exercise More' message – especially if they think they have successfully applied it to themselves – then they are less likely to question it. We focus on the diet successes – however short-term and misleading – and ignore the statistically greater number of failures.

All that explains why the debate has not moved forward for 40 years. Why we continue to push failure.

Now it is time to forget the prejudice, abandon the Hair Shirt Treatment, and look for changes that can really help.

PART 3: THE FUTURE

CHAPTER 12

The Future:
What Governments Can Do

"The people in power have created an obesity epidemic."
Robert Atkins

As Professor John Mathers of Newcastle University told The Guardian, "There's no point blaming individuals. We got into this mess because of the society we've created."

So, we need to change society – and not in a sneering, smug, look-at-me-with-my-spiralizer, kind of a way.

If there are wider trends to blame, then there are wider measures that can be effective. If there is a general trend, then there are general law changes and campaigns which can help.

Quite simply, there are things that governments can do to help their populations – but they have to be brave. They have to realise the 'Eat Less, Exercise More' message has failed and is irrelevant. They have to take on the Tiger that is the food and diet industry. If they accept the scale of obesity is the result of a changing society, then they can govern. Once they stop blaming individual laziness, then they can lead.

Lithuania, in 2018, is yet another example of a government backing away from potentially effective measures in order to 'work with the food industry' to find solutions. It is a bit like 'working with' a crocodile on their habit of eating other animals. There is a complete contradiction between genuinely tackling obesity – which means tackling sugar content, packaged food, processed food, sugary drinks, marketing and public information (basically everything that makes loads of money for a multi-billion pound series of businesses) – and cosying up to companies and their executives which are trying hard to protect their profits and their bonuses.

Harvard University's Susan Greenhalgh reported in 2019 about how the soda industry moved their efforts at influencing policy from the US to China.[61] Interviews with experts, along with trends in Government figures, "showed that from 1999 to 2015, China's obesity science and policy shifted markedly toward physical activity as Coca-Cola's influence in China increased. This shift aligned with Coca-Cola's message that it is activity, not diet, that matters—a claim few public health scholars accept. These changes correlated with the growing importance of Coca-Cola's funding, ideas, and affiliated researchers via ILSI-China (International Life Sciences Institute, US-based and corporate-funded). In putting its massive resources behind only one side of the science, and with no other parties sufficiently resourced to champion more balanced solutions that included regulation of the food industry, the company, working through ILSI re-directed China's chronic disease science, potentially compromising the public's health."

If somewhere as big, powerful, and independently-minded as China has joined the list of countries hoping to tame the Tiger, rather than control it, then that shows the scale of the task. The food industry is fighting hard to protect its empire. The job of governments is to stand up to that, just as once upon a time they had to be persuaded to stand up to the tobacco industry.

The first job of governments is to understand that they have a job to do. They can make a difference. Relying on the voluntary actions of the food industry is not enough. Then they have to hold their nerve; it may take a decade for the impact to become clear – maybe longer.

Nudge, nudge

In 2008, the book Nudge: Improving Decisions about Health Wealth and Happiness, written by University of Chicago economist Richard H. Thaler and Harvard Law School Professor Cass R. Sunstein, became popular with various politicians on both sides of the Atlantic. The book is based on older theories of psychotherapy, which look to find gentle ways of changing behaviour in specific groups of people. One of the most commonly quoted examples is painting the image of a housefly in the urinals at Schiphol Airport in Amsterdam to improve the aim of users.

It also takes account of Kahnemann's theory of System 1 and System 2 thinking, being targeted at the first, more instinctive, form of thinking. British Prime Minister David Cameron even set up a unit in No 10 Downing Street to look at ways of using this thinking at the heart of Government; predictably, it became known as the Nudge Unit.

Another common example of the theory is the idea of putting fruit and healthy food by the checkouts in shops, rather than sweets and chocolate as they tend to now. This theory had some success when tried by snack shops at Dutch train stations. However, it is worth remembering that most supermarkets put fresh produce by the entrance because we are more likely to buy something naughty – and more profitable – once we have something healthy in our trolley.

Nudge Economics definitely has some potential value, but its use is far from simple. We need a greater understanding. Also, it is particularly beloved by politicians because it is typically cheap to implement – which is not necessarily a recommendation.

Taxation is another way that governments can change behaviours.

Since October 2015, there has been a 5 pence charge for single-use plastic carrier bags in shops in England, following on from similar initiatives in Northern Ireland, Scotland, and Wales. Obviously, 5 pence per bag, on top of a £50 shop, is neither here nor there – loose change dropped down the side of a sofa – but the effect has been staggering. The UK Government estimates there has been a drop of 83% in the use of plastic bags since the change; that's going from around 140 bags for each person per year to around 25. Many of those still used are the result of online shopping deliveries, but further efforts are being made to reduce that number.

There were some fevered arguments against the charge before it was introduced gradually through Northern Ireland, Scotland, Wales, and England. For example, there were claims that shopping bags were themselves recycled as rubbish bags, so there was no point in the charge. WRAP (Waste and Resource Action Programme) studied the effect in Wales before and after the law changes, and concluded that bin liner sales did indeed go up as a result – but that increase cancelled out just 4% of the total drop in shop plastic bag usage. It shows how some fevered arguments can simply disappear from relevance after the event.

The bag 'tax' raises money, around £65million in England in 2016/17, but that is a side issue compared to the reduction of bags used. The fact that such a small charge can make such a big change shows why food and drink manufacturers are so scared of a Sugar Tax. Just as plastic bag usage has plummeted, they worry food and drink sales will fall substantially if the prices go up or the taste is less enticing. Just 5 pence per bag changed the mood, changed thought processes, and boosted something people wanted to do. It explains the vast amounts spent on lobbying, political donations, and dubious websites around the world that the food industry uses to fight sugar taxes.

That food and drink giants see sugar taxes as such a big threat strikes me as one of the best reasons for bringing them in.

Tax and bend

The message about sugar taxes is one some governments around the world have taken on board, although it is not easy to carry that through into policy changes. The prejudice against fat people can mean resentment about measures 'punishing' everyone for the greed of a few.

Also, the food industry spends huge amounts on lobbying and supporting political parties on all sides – they know which side their bread is buttered! Once again, prejudices against fat people help their lobbying. There are many measures around the world which have been tried and then abandoned under pressure; many more which have not even made it as far as becoming law.

The University of North Carolina, along with the Mexican Institute of Public Health, looked into the way a Sugar Tax was working in Mexico. The tax is roughly 4 cents per litre. It had the biggest impact on the poorest households, where the drop in purchases of sugary products was almost a third in 2015 – which is a good thing, of course.

This study contradicted a UNESDA (European food and drink industry) website claim there has been "No detectable impact on calorie intake or BMI." The University of Carolina study said, "Overall the result from our study contradicts industry reports of a decline in the effect of the tax after the first year of implementation." They added it was too early to measure the impact on obesity or public health. Just as losing weight over a short period through a diet is generally meaningless in the long-term, so these initiatives need to be measured over decades – seeing the effect on the next generation – before we jump to negative conclusions.

Adam Briggs of the Nuffield department of population health at Oxford University told The Guardian newspaper, the results were "really encouraging. The principle that price change leads to sustained behaviour change remains important." Some countries include high-intensity sweeteners in the tax, which I think is the right, evidence-based, way to go. Either way, if the change sees people from the poorer ends of society switch from soda to water, then – far from being penalised by the tax as UNESDA claim – they would save a fortune.

A report in Euromonitor International in December 2016 pointed out that 19 countries use taxes on sugary food and drinks, with more likely to follow. They estimate the positive impact in countries such as Mexico will increase if the tax is increased, One Peso per litre is too low, they argue. They also say the efforts could lead to a 20% reduction in worldwide sugar consumption, and talk about the significant tax revenues – hundreds of millions of Euros per year on average across

Europe – and higher levels of tax having a long-term effect in reducing intake.

Those who are addicted – needing a daily cola or chocolate bar, for example – will end up paying a little more. Where the tax could have a dramatic impact is at the other end of the scale – casual, or even careless, obesity – which I class as Lifestyle Obesity. It will steer people towards healthier and cheaper options, often before addiction can become an issue. On that basis, it is something which needs to be tried for 10-20 years before we have a real idea of how it is working.

Changing tax

The Organisation for Economic Co-operation and Development (OECD), produces an obesity update annually. Over the years, they have chronicled some of the efforts made by governments and noted where any impact has resulted. One example would be the Drink Up campaign in the US in 2013, spearheaded by Michelle Obama as chair of the Partnership for a Healthier America. Early data showed this had some success in increasing water drinking.

The widespread economic crisis of 2008 had a bad effect on food consumption around the world. For example, the OECD evidence shows households in the UK decreased food expenditure by almost 10%, but that meant the food they did buy was around 5% more calorific. Cheaper processed food tends to be more calorie-dense, and we know obesity is an issue which hits the poorer and less well-educated harder.

The report noted the advent of new sugar taxes in many countries, some at substantially higher rates. Such moves have met industry opposition, but the OECD says they were generally well received by the public. Denmark, Finland, France, and Hungary have applied their own tax measures, and the UK has started along that road. Public Health England released a 2018 report[62] just after the Sugar Tax had been introduced saying drinks manufacturers had reduced sugar in their products by 2% following the initial introduction of the tax, when PHE wanted to see a 20% decrease.

The Public Health Tax on food products in Hungary, in 2011, saw a 29% price increase, which led to a 27% drop in sales of those products. It has been estimated that 40% of food companies reformulated their products to take out or reduce the taxed ingredients, which is a win/win.

In Denmark, a tax on saturated fats resulted in people buying the same products in discount stores rather than high-priced supermarkets. Where that happened, of course, the effect on public health would have been limited. Political lobbying and controversy ultimately led to the measures being scrapped. It is fair to say fat is a much more ambiguous area than processed sugars.

France estimated a tax on sugary drinks would decrease consumption by 3.4 litres per person per year. Ireland's Department of Health estimated, in 2012, the impact would lead to a reduction of around 2,000 calories per person per week, leading to 10,000 fewer obese people. Nevertheless, those measures proved to be politically difficult, meaning the introduction of such a tax was delayed until 2018 in Ireland.

There is no international agreement on a level where sugar tax should apply; for example, it is set at 8 grams of sugar per 100 millilitres in the UK, and half that in South Africa.

Some sort of sugar tax seems a measure whose time has come after a period of fighting. I would support it strongly, which might surprise some people. I have two main reasons why I think it is an obvious move.

Firstly, some people, particularly children or their parents, will edge away from the more calorific choices. It will only be some of the time, but that is the first step towards reversing trends.

However, the second reason is the most important (though strangely it is often used as an argument against). Companies change the formulation of their food and drink to avoid a sugar tax. In many ways, that is the bigger goal.

It is used as an argument against because it means the tax produces less revenue than predicted – so it is not worth doing – even though the OECD evidence from around the world is that it still raises a substantial amount of the targeted revenue.

I would limit any sugar tax slightly and not put a tax on natural sugars, honey for instance, but definitely on refined sugars, High Fructose Corn, and so on. I would include high-intensity artificial sweeteners in the sugar tax because they create the need for sugar in the body regardless of whether they also provide it.

I would not tax fats because there is plenty of evidence that too many of them are actually helpful in health terms, though that approach could be refined to encourage the use of healthier fats. I mentioned earlier the dangers of low-fat products which use sugar to compensate. Just one last, small point about the potential revenue of a sugar tax – it may help reduce the stigma against fat people. So much of that is based on how much our 'greed' costs others; the tax may allow some perceptions to change because of the money raised.

Moving forward, someone needs to hold their nerve. Change needs clear vision and bravery, but there *are* measures that governments can take in terms of legislation and education which will change things for the better. If we hold governments to account, rather than individuals, then we can change the upward curve of the obesity graph.

Cooking up a storm

Governments would have to be firm against what would, no doubt, be a considerable storm whipped up by the drinks and food industries. When President Barack Obama brought in rules in the US about school meals, the food industry managed to get pizza added to the list of healthy foods because of the tomato content. At some point, we have to make a choice between big business and big people.

Here are some of the headline changes in advance of a UK Sugar Tax. In 2016 Tesco reduced their own brand soft drinks to less than 5 grams per 100 ml of sugar, to avoid the tax. "This is just one part of our plans to make the food on our shelves healthier by reducing levels of sugar, salt and fat in our own brands," Matt Davies, Tesco's chief executive for the UK and Republic of Ireland, told The Guardian.

"We have worked to make sure our soft drinks still taste great, just with less sugar. Tesco customers are now consuming on average over 20% less sugar from our soft drinks than in 2011. We're hoping this initiative will help make it a little easier for our customers to live more healthily."

Scottish soda drink manufacturer Irn-Bru also reformulated its traditional recipe to reduce sugar, though this led to petitions, protests, and stockpiling from customers who wanted to keep the old taste.

Lucozade Ribena Suntory committed to reformulating all their UK soft drink brands. "We are changing the complete portfolio," Dr. Naomi Grant, the company's director of research and development for GB and Ireland, told a Westminster Food and Nutrition Forum sugar reduction seminar. Food Manufacture magazine reported that her claim would lead to a 50% reduction in sugar.

Often reducing sugar levels means getting the flavour from more natural ingredients, which surely is part of the point. For instance, reducing the sugar in chocolate can be compensated for by increasing the cocoa. In other words, to improve chocolate, you add chocolate – which seems an obvious thing.

By way of response, there has been a classic misdirection strategy in place from the drinks companies, who prefer to focus on exercise and education instead of tax. A Sugar Tax was delayed on the Isle of Man with the promise of funds being used to educate people about exercise. Lucozade Ribena Suntory also looked to move the debate in that direction with a £30 million investment to get people exercising more.

That attempted deflection needs to be firmly ignored.

Perhaps the best examples for changing products in a positive way come from outside the soft drinks market, where artificial sweeteners are a worryingly obvious alternative.

Sugar – and salt, but that is a different debate for now – is a cheap way of making food more attractive. If the sugar content is going to be taxed, then the food manufacturers look at ways of maintaining the taste. Often that means replacing the sugar with better contents.

Sugar taxes are not going to end obesity overnight or raise enormous amounts of money. But if they reduce the overall sugar intake of a population, and increase the intake of more natural ingredients, then they will be a part of the answer.

Let fat people help themselves

There are some other simple things that governments can do which will help.

The first is to let fat people help themselves – no, not that way – by ensuring there is clear information provided on food packaging. There are so many misleading claims, appealing to the System 1 part of our brains; we can reduce obesity levels by giving people the chance to make clear and accurate decisions.

There is legislation about the information that needs to be given on the content labels of food packets, but it is usually in tiny writing tucked away on the back. Given the age profile of many overweight people, that is extremely hard to read. There is too much confusing information for simple decisions. While salt content, E numbers (generally just called the much less threatening 'flavouring'), and all the other bits of information are important to have available on the packet, they are not the most important piece of information.

Governments could make it law that there are two figures (at least one centimetre in size; once again size is important!) on the front of any packet. One is the total number of calories in the packet; the other is the number of calories per 100 grams. It would be the food equivalent of the message on the side of cigarette packets about health dangers. Once we know those two pieces of information, we can make up our own minds.

There needs to be an awareness that calories are only part of the story; for instance, there is a huge difference between 100 calories of corn on the cob and 100 calories of High Fructose Corn syrup. However, the figure would at least provide an indication.

There is very little real-world research on this issue; much of what has been done has either taken place on university campuses or been low level. In 2018, the Cochrane Report,[63] produced by scientists across a range of British universities, suggested that available research supported the idea that people reduced their calorie intake by a little under 10% if calories were on the menu when eating out.

In the US, chains with more than 20 outlets have to show calorie numbers, an Obama administration move which was fiercely fought by the food industry until 2018. For example, cinema chains fought against showing 1,000 calories in their packs of popcorn. However, one side effect of the ruling could be product changes to avoid such scary numbers.

When Seattle restaurants were made to put nutritional information on their menus in 2009, the calories, salt content and saturated fat contents of the food served all improved.[64]

I would simply say that information is king. Often, we make decisions in ignorance, and I have little doubt there would be a positive impact on both the recipes and our choices if such policies were implemented more widely.

Self-serving

There is plenty of space for nutritional numbers on packaging; there's no problem at all putting them there because, at the moment, the food companies put different, more confusing claims there. They pick on potential health benefits which may or may not be fully accurate; even if they are true, they may not be the whole truth.

Most annoyingly, food companies find space to tell you how many calories there are per serving, which is the most useless and misleading piece of information around. Here is a genuine conversation I had recently. "You shouldn't eat that pasta salad and think it's healthy, because it's full of calories," I said. "It's only 200 calories for half a pack, that's not bad," came the reply. But in small letters, written at right angles to the main claim about 200 calories *"per serving,"* it says that figure applies to one-sixth of the carton. In fact, the pasta salad contains 600 calories for half, 1,200 calories in total. It shows the power of marketing – we automatically think of 'their' serving sizes are the same as 'our' serving sizes and do the maths from there.

Take one breakfast cereal which promised a little more than 100 calories per serving. Read the small print, and it says those figures are for 17 servings per small box. I would finish a box in three or four servings.

It is hard to believe there is anyone in the country who ever got 17 separate breakfasts out of that box. I'm not sure a hamster would get that many meals out of it. They should be made to say there are around 2,000 calories in the box and let us work out the rest.

Remember the System 1 thinking test when people were asked to decide how much to offer for a bottle of champagne, and how people were manipulated by the apparently random number pulled out of the bag beforehand? Well, calories per serving act in the same way; give us a low number to start with, and we can be manipulated. That is why we need the government to step in on our side.

If you see two breakfast cereals and one has 3,000 calories in big numbers on the front, and the other has 1,500, then you will make better decisions more often.

Another area for attention is clearly the advertising of junk food. In the UK, many of the arguments have focused on children and the impact of advertising before 9pm. Indeed, Public Health England, among many others, have argued for a total ban on such TV adverts before that time.

Of course, the food industry argues against, saying the adverts have little impact and banning them would restrict personal choice. These companies are extremely professional; they analyse the impact of every advert they spend money on in order to maximise best practice and target their cash more effectively. The fact they continue to advertise means, by definition, those adverts have an impact on their bottom line. That alone is a reason for looking to ban them. In many ways, the current debate is reminiscent of the smoking ban in public places or charging people for carrier bags in shops. Before those policies came in, they were controversial; afterwards, many people wondered what the fuss was about. Both have been highly effective in achieving their objectives.

Control advertising, ban calories per serving as an advertised measurement, enforce clear information for total calories and calories per 100g on packaging and menus. It's fairly simple, really. So, *there are* things governments can do to help their populations. The first step is to understand this is not only something they *can* do, but something they have a responsibility *to do*. This means ignoring the arguments from the food industry, particularly those that frame obesity in terms of control and exercise. The obesity sweeping the world is clearly a wider trend and governments need to take wider action to combat it.

CHAPTER 13

The Future 2:
What Science Can Do

"We can't solve problems by using the same kind of thinking we used when we created them."

Albert Einstein

The BBC TV programme The Right Diet for You did an experiment. They looked at the stomach hormone levels of a group of overweight people, then offered them a wide variety of food from a constantly rotating sushi bar. They predicted in advance who would eat the most, based on those hormone tests, hypothesizing that the highest levels of hunger hormones would lead to the greatest amount of food consumed.

Hey Presto, it turned out those predictions were pretty accurate – the people with the highest level of hunger hormones were indeed the people who ate the most.

Just as my mind was wandering towards the toilet habits of bears in the woods, the religious persuasion of the Pope, and the rotational swimming of one-legged ducks, came the surprise.

They announced this test had never been done before.

Really?

More than $800 million a year is spent on obesity research in the US alone, whilst UK figures run well into the double figures of millions of pounds. It is estimated that treating obesity costs the National Health Service, in the UK, more than £4bn a year; a figure that can be inflated to more than £5bn or £6bn depending on the level of fat-beating you want to get into. Estimates in the United States put the annual cost at between $150-200 billion. Meanwhile, consultancy firm McKinsey has estimated the global cost of obesity at $2 trillion – only smoking, war, and terror cost more. Given the scale of the potential reward, it is a shame the vast majority of that research is focused on irrelevances.

It took a TV programme – a one-off test on a small sample – to even scratch the surface on what seems to me the most obvious area of research. The obsession with diets and the willpower myth, along with reinforced messages as to the dangers of being fat, has meant the most promising area of research has been almost completely ignored. We are back to so-called experts not believing fat people, not listening to us, preferring to do experiments on rats rather than following what we have to say about why we are fat. Everything fat people say has been painted as an excuse for far too long.

These scientists are the tourists abroad who shout loudly instead of learning the language. At the very least, that example from a TV programme is a piece of research which should be repeated on a bigger and more scientific scale to test the findings fully.

At the time of writing, there is a team at Imperial College, London, looking into the impact of stomach hormones on addiction in the areas of obesity, smoking, alcohol, and gambling. Their research could be a first step towards realistic explanations and answers. At least they are looking in the right direction.

Skinny genes

"It is a lottery. We inherit these genes, and they either may contribute to a higher tendency to gain weight or even may protect you from gaining weight. So, it is not really about people's fault; it is actually about understanding there is a lottery.

"We can modify some things in our own environment, but to understand there is actually a real biology underlying it, this is really important."

Not my words, but those of Cambridge University Professor Sadaf Farooqi, of the Department of Clinical Biochemistry, Cambridge Institute for Medical Research, speaking to the BBC's Truth About Obesity programme.

We need to accept we are what we are. We need to concentrate on realistic goals which will impact positively on our health and – possibly – our weight.

When asked if weight gain was as simple as not going to the gym, drinking more beers, and eating badly, Professor Farooqi replied, "If you do all those things, you are likely to gain weight, but there will be other people just like you who are also doing those things who will not gain weight. The reason why you might, is linked to your genes."

Farooqi and her team have identified around 100 gene mutations which affect 40-70% of our weight. One mutated gene, MC4R, gives us almost no chance of avoiding obesity, but it only affects around 1% of people. As for the rest of us, we may have some or all of those mutations, but the likelihood is that we have all sorts of different mixes.

The biggest area affected by these genes is leptin production and leptin receptors (the body's system for telling us we are full). If that message is not sent, or not received, then we are more likely to want more and become overweight.

Why is this important when plotting a way forward? Because we have to understand ourselves first of all – *then* we can work out what will help each of us.

It tallies with the research by Dr. Kevin Hall which followed the participants of The Biggest Loser, that there is a partially pre-determined level of weight for all of us; for better or for worse. Everyone focuses on the weight lost in diets, not the weight put back on afterwards in most cases. We have to acknowledge both to find real answers.

In 2018, Kings College, London, carried out the world's largest investigation trying to identify the gene variations which lead to depression. The researchers came up with 44, including 30 new ones. That is a small part of the total picture around depression, but has started the process of focusing research on anti-depressant drugs which may have a better chance of working. A similarly detailed level of knowledge about the genes which may lead to obesity would also be incredibly useful.

Gut reactions

It has taken a long time for science to get around to examining areas which could be deemed an 'excuse' for fat people, or areas which could result in non-punishing, hair-shirt solutions. Yet the more we can look at new explanations for obesity, the more we can look for new – and more realistic – solutions.

A few studies have started to find substantial links between microbiome in the stomach guts and obesity. The microbiome is the combination of microbes that convert food into energy in our stomachs – bacteria, viruses, fungi, and a whole host of tiny micro-organisms. The balance is a combination of nature and nurture; in other words, some inherited and some as a result of our environment.

Increasingly this area is being seen as important as genetics, in terms of influencing our bodies. It seems obvious to say the way they impact our food intake is crucial to the amount of energy we may end up storing as fat. It also affects appetite, both initial urges and when we feel full. The way people react differently to various foods is explained by this.

"Whether tomatoes are good or bad for you, whether rice is good for you or worse for you than ice cream, and so on, is explained by your microbiome. For obesity, different kinds of microbes are involved in the differences between lean and obese humans," human microbiome expert Rob Knight, Professor of Paediatrics, Computer Science and Engineering at the University of California San Diego, told The Guardian in 2018.

Researchers at Lund University, in Sweden, have added evidence to the link[65] to both obesity and Type 2 diabetes, amongst other areas such as cardiovascular disease. Part of their research involved studying the bacterial content of poo, so you feel they deserved to come up with something worthwhile from their research.

They focused on the metabolites in our blood, which means the substances which help our activities and metabolism such as lactic acid and antibiotics (to give just a couple of the better-known examples.) Basically, they dictate how much food we want, how well we take energy from food in the first place, and then how efficiently we use it. In other words, pretty much everything!

They found 19 different metabolites connected to obesity. Two in particular, glutamate and BCAA (branched-chain and aromatic amino acids, since you ask) had the strongest connections. In turn, those metabolites were linked to four particular bacteria in the gut. "The differences in BMI were largely explained by the differences in the levels of glutamate and BCAA. This indicates that the metabolites and gut bacteria interact, rather than being independent of each other. This means that future studies should focus more on how the composition of gut bacteria can be modified to reduce the risk of obesity and associated metabolic diseases and cardiovascular disease," Marju Orho-Melander, Professor of Genetic Epidemiology at Lund University, told Science Daily.

Gut microbes are also being linked to depression, and even how well we cope with cancer treatment. Researchers say the sooner we have large scale studies to find what a base-level, healthy gut consists of, then the sooner we can identify anomalies and look to use that information to bring change. It would help to explain the link between pollution and obesity for example, and certain food types and obesity; the list can be pretty lengthy.

It is a highly promising area because it may be easier to influence our gut microbiome than our genetics.

A whole new holistic approach needed

We rely on science to help get us out of this obesity crisis, but there are two problems with the way science happens. The first is that, as scientists progress, their areas of specialisation get narrower and narrower. This approach was typified by one professor who criticised people's laziness as a factor in rising rates of diabetes, which was his area of research. However, when asked if this laziness was the result of the chemistry of the brain, he replied that was not his area of expertise. That is how science works – people end up in silos of specialism.

Scientists have largely abandoned the holistic approach, leaving that field free for charlatans. It is not a good combination.

Too much research is concentrated on finding out all the bad consequences of being fat, in the hope that will persuade fat people to see sense. I don't know how to put this more simply. Nothing – no report, no scaremongering, no fear of the future – will ever be worse than the day-to-day existence of being fat.

So, I would scrap every single research project worldwide aimed at showing how bad obesity is for us. The only success for those research projects is to make thin people smugger – if that's possible – certainly they have all patently failed to tackle obesity effectively.

There is a second problem with the way science works. Understandably enough it relies on bright people, highly-qualified people, ambitious people. People who are looking to move onward and upward in their careers. They don't mind a bit of number crunching, but repetitive experiments for more than a decade is pretty low down on their Personal Life Plans.

Keeping a team of academics together for longer than five years, working on the same project, is hard to fund. As a result, many studies are short-term, one or two years, often the eight months of an academic year or shorter. Also, far too many of those research projects are funded by the food industry – and it is amazing in all walks of life just how many research projects back up the views of the people who fund them. In her 2018 book Unsavory Truth: how food companies skew the science of what we eat, New York University Professor Marion Nestle says that out of 168 food and drink industry-funded studies she looked at when trying to find unbiased examples, only 12 did not have favourable results for the funders.

In other words, the system of scientific research is almost set up to fail in the area of obesity where trends can take place over many decades. It is no surprise that many of the people quoted in this book are professors who have dedicated large chunks of their lives to this study. It is another reason why the experiences of fat people over decades should be taken more seriously. We have long-term experiences that most of the scientists are missing.

Index-linked

Another area where scientists have helped to maximise the scale of the problem – and therefore where they can help to defuse the hysteria – is BMI.

I have already gone into why the Body Mass Index is such an imperfect measure (the change of what constituted a healthy BMI was arbitrary and based on out-of-date figures). It helped increase the focus on obesity when the World Health Organisation dubbed it a worldwide epidemic, and that change certainly did no harm to the careers of those in the diet and nutrition industry.

But it makes no sense at all to have a 'healthy BMI' that does not include the healthiest weight. While the single healthiest weight in terms of life expectancy is 27, the best range for men is 25-28 – which is in the overweight category of BMI. While being chubby is better for you than being a marathon runner, it seems mad to demonise that group. The healthiest weight range for women is a BMI of 21-28.

When Usain Bolt, at his athletic peak as the fastest man on the planet, only squeezes into the healthy BMI bracket by 0.1, then surely something needs to be recognised as wrong.

But there is another side to the figures. If we do increase the healthy BMI range to something more realistic and which tallies with the figures of modern society, then we reduce the hysteria around obesity. It would allow us to stop panicking, stop blaming, and start focusing on what will help.

BMI is a rotten index. It would be a good start if scientists recognised that, and changed official figures as a result; it would be even better if they found a new way of calculating how we are overweight and by how much. There are many current research projects which use methods other than BMI to quantify those taking part.

The lessons of smoking

We need to make a decision between what *really* works – and what we think *should* work. They are usually two very different things. Continual warnings about the dangers of being fat have not worked, nor is there any evidence they ever will. There are lessons to be learned from what has (and has not) worked in terms of reducing smoking numbers on a large scale.

After 40 years of negative messages and high taxes having a gradual impact, recently the number of smokers in the UK dropped dramatically to the lowest levels since World War II.

So, what has changed? The health risks of smoking have been generally known and understood since the 1970s. While some in the older generations started smoked believing it was actually good for them, every single one of the hundreds of smokers I have known has fully realised they were damaging their own health to some extent. That health message has been driven home through hard-hitting advertising campaigns, and new and ever-stronger wording on cigarette packets; but all to little avail.

If you are looking for the reasons why the statistics are changing more rapidly now, then you need to look at factors which have changed recently. It turns out there has been a double-pronged attack in terms of technology and policy.

The technology is vaping – inhaling the vapour of an electronic cigarette. Now vaping is controversial and has its own negative impacts; it still involves inhaling nicotine after all, some consider it a gateway to smoking, and it also includes some cancer-causing chemicals (but at much lower levels than cigarettes). In fact, there is plenty of research to show it is clearly better than smoking, but worse than giving up completely. Vaping is 95% better than smoking, according to Public Health England. However, my point is about the reaction.

Statistically, vaping or nicotine patches or nicotine chewing gum are more successful in helping people give up smoking compared to giving up with no help. The American Cancer Society estimates the success of going cold turkey at 4-7%. There are more than 150 studies which show that nicotine replacement therapies, in some form or another, improves the chances of giving up by 50-70%.

But vaping is about more than nicotine; it has offered an additional step forward. Vaping provides a nicotine hit, and it also satisfies the physical habit of smoking. The hold-it-in-your-hand, take-it-to-your-lips physical action that is ingrained through smoking is also satisfied. In a way, it gives the mind and entrenched behavioural habits some support.

Anecdotally, people are more likely to be congratulated socially for going cold turkey rather than embracing one of the softer – and more successful – options, but that is another story for now.

That's the technological change. At the same time, there have been changes to the law in terms of where and when you can smoke. The workplace and public places have become out of bounds.

Smoking has become much harder and much less socially acceptable thanks to the ban on smoking in public buildings. Suddenly smokers have been banished to stand outside offices, pubs, and public transport. It makes it much more difficult and, depending on the weather, potentially unpleasant. The smell that surrounds smokers has also become more noticeable than ever to non-smokers who are likely to strengthen their own stance on what is acceptable and where. Of course, that does not stop the hardened smoker, but it does influence those on the edges, or at least reduce their intake slightly.

The ban started because of the dangers of 'passive smoking' and the health risks for non-smokers in a smoky environment. There were successful lawsuits. In order to head these off, measures were brought in to prevent passive smoking risks, and that meant not being able to smoke in enclosed public areas.

In simple terms, those changes mean that smoking is harder to do than it used to be and, by extension, it is easier to give up than it used to be. The double-pronged attack has been far more successful than decades of public information campaigns about the dangers of smoking, combined with punitive taxes.

People still smoke, the battle is not won, but the numbers have dropped across the board and hopefully will continue to do so.

It is a blueprint for encouraging weight loss. The approach which has had the most limited success with smokers is still the preferred option, for many, for dealing with weight loss. The messages in public information, publications, and social media are mostly that fat people should choose the hard route rather than being offered an easier method. I believe the easier we can make it, the better.

Finding an equivalent to the ban on smoking in public places would be a government matter, dealt with in the previous chapter. However, finding a food equivalent of vaping is certainly an area where scientific research could work.

The central thrust would be to find out what works in terms of triggering our brains and the body's hormones either to restrict appetite in the first place or to make us feel full earlier. Which foods make us feel the fullest per calorie? How can we trigger those full feelings for longer? Is there an easy way of stimulating those feelings without extra calories? What balance of food satisfies our cravings over a period of years? How can we change our diets for years to come, not just weeks or months?

Just as with smoking, we need to start accepting softer and more successful solutions rather than the most punishing and least effective. It would make listening to fat people a perfectly respectable form of research, which in turn would save a fortune and make life more pleasant for millions of rats!

Bariatric surgery

Bariatric surgery seems, at first glance, a really ignorant solution to obesity – a surgical reduction in stomach capacity to limit food intake. The public perception of the principle behind it relies on prejudice against fat people being greedy so and so's. Reduce the size of their stomachs and see them trying to stuff their faces then!

In reality, the origins of the surgery, which has been around since the 1950's, is slightly different. The first efforts were not particularly successful with plenty of side effects. However, in 1966, University of Iowa surgeon Dr. Ed Mason, along with his colleague Dr. Chikashi Ito, noticed that patients who had part of their stomach taken out because of cancer also went on to lose a lot of weight. It was that cause and effect which led to the development of bariatric surgery, not prejudice.

Removing a chunk of stomach is still the most common surgery for obesity, but there are other similar approaches such as a gastric bypass (using a ring to limit the size of the stomach) and the gastric balloon (which expands inside the stomach to limit capacity) in use. All bariatric surgery means a big and expensive operation, although there have been attempts to produce pills which have the same effect by expanding in the stomach without surgery.

There are problems with bariatric surgery, ranging from the possibility of dying on the operating table, or shortly afterwards, through to feeling a little bit sick occasionally. However, there is often substantial short-term weight loss and a good long-term prognosis in terms of sustaining most, if not all, of that weight loss for some people.

Karen Synne Groven, of the University of Oslo in Norway, has done a series of studies which show both sides of bariatric surgery. Social and physical issues creep in over a period of time, not least that it is really hard to eat healthily. Loss of energy is a significant factor for around a fifth of the people she studied in depth. She also found there is a reluctance of people to look for these negative stories following bariatric surgery – and also a reluctance from those who had gone through it to reveal the problems.

Of course, bariatric surgeons and societies push the long-term success, and indeed it does seem to be the most effective long-term solution in a physical sense.

The public focus is on the physical changes, basically the idea that it prevents someone being greedy. I am much more interested in the behavioural changes, in terms of a reduction of hunger and feeling full more easily.

The surgery has an impact on the stomach hormones in many people; however, some people do not experience a reduction in hunger urges and sometimes that causes ongoing problems – effectively breaking the surgery to get back towards previous capacity. UK figures from 2017 showed that roughly 1 in 15 of the surgeries needed to be revised. It is not as simple as reducing the size of the stomach to lose weight; it seems it does not work unless it triggers a hormonal change. Where it works, the surgery changes the levels of hormones such as ghrelin, GIP, GLP and PYY – the gut hormones which communicate with the hunger centres of the brain.

Part of me wonders whether bariatric surgery is actually barking up the wrong tree; success has little to do with stomach reduction and much more to do with the hormonal changes. I know from personal experience that after an operation which had nothing to do with the stomach, it was easy to lose weight for a period of time. I found weight loss much easier for a year or so, on two separate occasions. Many of the changes in terms of diabetes and hunger levels are immediate in some people, therefore the result of the surgical process rather than the long-term result of the surgery.

If there is a way of changing the levels of hormones without changing the size of the stomach, then that would allow for much healthier long-term nutrition and a more positive relationship with food.

More research needs to be done on whether those effects can be replicated in other ways, or through less dramatic surgery. Bariatric surgery is not a perfect solution but it does seem – for some people – at least to be a solution.

What's in a word?

The Eskimos famously have more than 53 words for snow, and the various types of snow they come across. The Sami people, who live in Northern Scandinavia and Russia, have at least 180 words for snow and ice. Interestingly, they have more than 1,000 words for various types of reindeer down to some very personal physical distinctions such as the size of a bull's testicles.

Yet we have one word for fat. The oily substance in our bodies, the layer under our skin, fatty acids of various types, the overall appearance – we use one word to cover all sorts of very different things.

Dictionary.com has 22 distinct meanings for the word fat, with another five idioms such as 'chewing the fat' added on. A similar umbrella word for fat exists in many Western languages.

Why is this a problem? Well, the overall impression of the word is bad, so it means everything gets wrapped up under that negative perception. But some fats are not only good, they are *essential* for our survival; they play a key part in a healthily-balanced diet and can even play a key part in weight loss. There are good fats and bad fats; calling them the same thing does not help the debate or our understanding.

For instance, we know the oily fat of many fish is good for us, and the same goes for good quality olive oil. Omega 3 and Omega 6 fats are important – especially to keep in them in balance. We are getting the message that avocado is good for us precisely because it is full of fats, but overall the message in relation to fat is confused at best.

The word seems to be a barrier to differentiating good from bad. Even where there are clear scientific studies showing the benefits of some fats in reducing the risk of diabetes, to take one example, there is reluctance to make those recommendations official. Governments are reluctant to recommend fats – even when they should.

So, one thing scientists can do is to come to some consensus about good and bad fats and provide some clearer recommendations. There was a clear scientific consensus against the Atkins Diet because it contained too much fat, now there is an equally clear view that the right kinds of fat can indeed have a beneficial influence on weight loss. If we can distinguish between them more clearly, then maybe that will help.

Low-fat foods are considered good when in reality many are much worse for us than the natural fat originals, both in terms of health and obesity.

A lesson can be learned from the debate and usage around the word 'gender' – which is, after all, another area largely governed by genetics and hormones. Gender differences in human beings have existed as long as the hills; changing the language has been a clear start in the process of changing attitudes. Hence transgender, agender, bigender, cisgender, gender fluid, gender identity, gender non-conforming, gender straight, gender queer, gender variant, and third gender; just some of the words including 'gender.' Thesafezoneproject lists no fewer than 90 words associated with forms of sexuality and behavior.

The scientists can help in finding a clearer consensus of what fats are good and helpful, and they can help in breaking down the prejudices against good fats – but maybe the linguists are needed, as well, to find better ways of changing the language. I will give the process a nudge by throwing my weight behind 'Superfats' as a description for all the good fats, 'Bad fats' for the rest. Many would potentially include Low Fat in this second category.

Is there an anti-hunger drug?

There are anti-obesity drugs available, both on prescription and through the Wild West of the online world. The latter range from drugs which will kill you to pills which will be of no help at all. The online world is tempting as it offers easy answers, but it is best ignored completely. Suffice it to say, if there were a genuine solution to the obesity crisis, marketeers would not need to send spam emails!

You can get drugs prescribed on the NHS, but they work on attracting the fat molecules in food so you digest less fat in the stomach. They have a relatively low success rate. My own doctor mentioned their existence in the most half-hearted way imaginable and I was happy to agree there were better ways of approaching the issue. We know the body can adjust, getting sugar from carbohydrates to make up for the disappointment of low-calorie soda for instance. Also, given what we have discovered about the health benefits of natural fats, these pills may even be counter-productive. Maybe they are based around the confusion over the word more than anything else. Once again, they are not worth considering as a widespread answer.

However, there is one interesting possibility which needs a lot more scientific research.

There is a drug called Nalmefene which is prescribed on the NHS in the UK for alcohol dependence, which has also been tried in the areas of gambling and opioid addiction. An equivalent was available in the US for opioid overdoses, but it was expensive and did not sell well. It has never been used in the US for the other areas, such as alcohol.

Nalmefene works on the opioid receptors of the brain, the same areas that get triggered by both heroin and food. It also acts as a dopamine suppressant, which means it limits reward-motivated behaviour. An example would be how a second glass of wine gives certain people's brains a chemical boost. This drug is aimed at switching off that desire.

A radio interview gave a clue about one reason why there has been so little research in this area. The questioner asked: how does it work. The scientist's reply was that the person has a glass or two of wine, for instance, and then stops wanting another drink. So, do they feel sick, or nauseous, to put them off? No, they just stop wanting more. How about a headache or sickness? No, they just stop wanting more.

The questions about bad side effects went on, but the interview illustrated the central problem with understanding addiction. There is no appetite for a drug which just works; there is a desire for a drug which works by punishing. Nalmefene has passed enough tests to show it works in enough cases to be an option in the treatment of alcoholism in the UK. However, it may be better suited for lower levels of intake which tend not to require medical intervention.

Nalmafene does not work for food intake but finding a food equivalent would be a massive breakthrough. One drug which was hailed by Britain's National Obesity Forum's Tam Fry as a potential "Holy Grail" of weight loss is Lorcaserin. It seems it may work as an appetite suppressant for some people.

It has been available in the US since 2013 as Belviq, and costs between $200-300 per month. It has been found by the Harvard associated Brigham and Women's Hospital to have no negative impact on heart problems – such side effects having been considered a serious risk of previous drugs. The research has shown that slightly more than double the number of participants lost more than 5% of their starting weight (39% compared to 17%) for Lorcaserin compared to a placebo.

Once again the study only lasted 12 months, so the long-term – five to ten year – impact is still in doubt. As obesity expert Professor Jason Halford, of Liverpool University, told The Daily Telegraph, "We don't have any appetite suppressants available on the NHS. We have a massive great gap between lifestyle modification and surgery."

At least this research seems to be moving in a positive direction. The process of moving, albeit slowly, towards a hormonal approach to obesity is not dissimilar to our growing understanding of depression as an uncontrolled change of brain chemicals and hormones. Our increased understanding has led to anti-depressant pills that try to fight that chemical imbalance, backed up by new research that anti-depressants really do help in the majority of cases. It should encourage us to go further down this road in the fight against obesity.

What's in our food

Whilst researching this book, I have found so many ways in which scientific research is at odds to our common beliefs about obesity. Those doubts also stretch to parts of the scientific community. There is a desire to dismiss the reports which do not tie in with our prejudices against fat people.

Time and time again, research I find interesting is dismissed by others – but not through picking holes in the theory. Usually, the dismissive arguments are that the research group was too small, or the timescale too short, but these are not followed by bigger samples being studied over a longer period of time if the premise is not popular.

So, we have research which shows natural fats are important in the fight against diabetes. We know the majority of diet drinks are consumed by obese people, but no detailed research exists as to why that is a bad thing. We have research showing the benefits of dark chocolate or natural cocoa, some funded by the chocolate industry. We have research showing the long-term benefits of having chocolate cake for breakfast. We have research showing there is no health negative in butter, but a 4% drop in diabetes rates.

These are lots of areas which offer attainable solutions for marginally improving health rates. We know diabetes rates have rocketed in an era of increasing low-fat food and reduced butter consumption. They may or may not be connected – just statistical correlations – but we have accepted similar links between obesity and other areas of health just because these things are happening at the same time.

Why is it so hard to come up with a scientific consensus in these areas? You have eminent scientists arguing, for example, about the substantial health benefits of natural fats. The case seems pretty convincing on a theoretical level and in terms of study results, with a multitude of research projects all around the world available. So why is this not accepted? Or at the very least, why is there little or no recent evidence to the contrary; studies that are better researched on more people over a longer period of time?

There is a deep problem with scientific funding which goes far wider than just obesity research. In her book, How Economics Shapes Science, Georgia State Economics Professor Paula Stephan analyses how research in popular areas is more likely to get funding and also to lead to further jobs for the scientists involved. With the increasingly competitive world of scientific research depending so heavily on governments and commercial funding, there is a strong push towards safe areas of research and safe answers. It is harder than ever to get funding to swim against the tide.

Fear of failure

There is one more way in which the scientific community has let us down in terms of obesity research. They have a fear of failure, or more accurately a fear of studying failure.

Much of the focus of science in the area of obesity has been on what helps people lose weight. Inevitably, that means focusing on the short-term and/or the unusual.

We know that more than 80% of people who lose weight in diets will put that weight (and often more) back on over the next four years and more. The focus of research is either on how they lost that weight in the

150

first place (ignoring the future failure), or it concentrates on the 20% who maintain lost body weight.

If people succeed in losing weight for the long-term, my first question would be about how they put on weight in the first place. If they are physically thin people who slipped into an unhealthy lifestyle, which was easy enough to change, then the lessons are only applicable to others like them. Rather than studying that group, I would exclude them. They are potentially just different to the other 80%, not examples to follow.

In Matthew Syed's book, Black Box Thinking, which was mentioned earlier in this book, he looks at how certain areas of knowledge progress through the study of failure, while others stagnate because of a desire to cover up failure. Aviation learns and moves forward, compared with many examples in the health world where advancement has been slower or not happened at all.

It is a really interesting comparison because, of course, no-one looks at the failures in obesity, nobody looks at the people who put on weight and asks *why*. We look at the people who have lost weight and think they are potentially the norm, when all the figures show they are a tiny minority.

If we looked at all the people who did not lose weight, who put it on, and did sympathetic research over a period of time, then we could move the debate forward far more effectively.

What could people have changed? What were the areas that made a difference? What were the triggers in terms of bullying, being ignored for jobs, or relationship issues? What were the key foods; were they takeaways or packaged meals, for instance? What were the habits? What could be done better?

Studying the successes of the dieting world has not helped at all, so perhaps studying the failures with sympathy would work better. It would mean ditching the rats and listening to fat people, but hey ho, you can't have everything.

To sum up, scientists have to start listening to, and believing, fat people. *Far greater* research should be geared towards changing the pattern of hunger hormones, as pleasant solutions are more likely to work than punishing ones.

Changes to the microbiome may well provide a cheap and easy key to success. Faecal transplants, or taking the best parts of what has been dubbed "Super Poo" from a healthy donor, has become a common and effective way of boosting people's microbiome to combat a variety of stomach illnesses and conditions. Maybe something similar, using the stomach hormones of someone who deals with food efficiently, may be a promising avenue of research.

I keep coming back to the periods after knee operations when I simply was not hungry. I could eat what I liked because I only wanted smaller quantities. It was heaven in every way – and I also lost weight. It was not a conscious decision, it was not willpower or a diet; it was just a different feeling.

If science can find a way of re-creating that feeling, then we will take a massive step forward in solving the obesity crisis.

CHAPTER 14

The Future 3:
I Believe The Children
Are Our Future

"**Childhood obesity isn't some simple, discrete issue. There's no one cause we can pinpoint. There's no one program we can fund to make it go away. Rather, it's an issue that touches on every aspect of how we live and how we work.**"

Michelle Obama

While the problems of adult obesity are serious, perhaps the area of greatest expansion has been in childhood obesity. There is plenty of research that diseases such as diabetes are more common in younger people, but you only have to open your eyes and look around to realise this is a growing issue.

It is vitally important for two reasons. Firstly, the increase in the size of many children is a serious health issue, in itself ,in the short-term. Secondly – and perhaps more importantly – these are the adults of the future. We know it is really hard to lose weight in later life, so the longer we can delay any gains the better.

It is also worth remembering that children's metabolisms cover up a variety of sins – you only have to think of the age-old battle with parents trying to get their child to wear an extra layer to know they cope with the cold better. Children are also lighter, by definition, and naturally more active.

However, they will become adults, and it is pretty unlikely they will get smaller. Even if they are not fat children, bad habits can catch up with them in later life. All too often, children are writing the obesity cheques that they will pay as adults. Some children become overweight, others do not, but both groups may be storing up problems with unhealthy lifestyles.

That is why, although there is a massive emphasis on childhood obesity, there is a wider problem than children who are overweight. It is about sowing good habits early which they will carry through life – whether or not they are overweight.

The UK Government estimates that nearly a third of children aged 2-15 are overweight or obese. Ignoring, for now, doubts over the reliability of BMI for those statistics, there is clearly a problem. They also estimate children are getting obese younger, and that the biggest problems stem from children from poorer backgrounds; by the age of 11, children from the poorest income groups are three times more likely to be obese compared to well-off peers.[66]

In the US, the problem appears to have plateaued at high levels of around 17%, or 12.7 million children, between the ages of 2-19 years-old.[67] Once again, the problem is significantly bigger in lower-income households. Apart from the obvious dietary causes, researchers have highlighted increased birth weight leading to a propensity for obesity in later life, lack of breastfeeding in the first six months, and childhood illnesses such as asthma and diarrhoea.

In 2016, the World Health Organisation estimated that there were 41 million children under the age of five considered to be obese, with almost half of them living in Asia and a quarter in Africa – where the numbers more than doubled between 1990 and 2013.

It is not surprising that areas you might associate with poverty have been badly hit. Research by the Food Foundation think tank in the UK estimated, in 2018, that the poorest 20% of families would need to spend 40% of their income on food to eat healthily. They calculated around 4 million people in the UK live in households which cannot afford to buy enough healthy foods – fruit, vegetables, fish and so on – to meet official recommendations.

Poverty represents potential for the food manufacturers. It provides the opportunity to sell cheap, processed, filling, energy-dense food that will satisfy people for less money than a bag of organic carrots. It makes Asia, Africa, and South America particular targets for commercial expansion.

As The New York Times reported, Nestle has created a network of door-to-door vendors in Brazil to sell their products which makes them an essential part of the economic fabric in poor areas. Childhood obesity is a major issue in these areas, but healthier eating could increase poverty in the short-term because of losing the jobs Nestle have created. The 2017 report by Andrew Jacobs and Matt Richtel said, "Nestlé's direct-sales army in Brazil is part of a broader transformation of the food system that is delivering Western-style processed food and sugary drinks to the most isolated pockets of Latin America, Africa and Asia. As their growth slows in the wealthiest countries, multinational food companies like Nestlé, PepsiCo and General Mills have been aggressively expanding their presence in developing nations, unleashing a marketing juggernaut that is upending traditional diets from Brazil to Ghana to India."

We've been Ad

One of the key battlegrounds in the fight against junior obesity has been trying to restrict advertising aimed at children. The facts and figures are concerning, to say the least.

Heart Foundation-funded research at the University of Adelaide in Australia showed junk food ads are shown more on TV at times when children are watching. Professor Lisa Smithers found children watch twice the amount of unhealthy food advertising as healthy food advertising; more than 800 adverts per year if they watch 80 minutes of TV a day.

"The World Health Organization has concluded that food marketing influences the types of foods that children prefer to eat, ask their parents for, and ultimately consume," added Professor Smithers.

Nielsen, a global information and measurement company, estimated the average figures in the US are 32 hours of TV a week for children aged 2-5 (four-and-a-half hours a day), 28 hours a week for children 6-8 (four hours a day). In the 8-18 age bracket, social media and internet also play a key role; the total for internet activity and TV is estimated at four-and-a-half hours a day. That means that youngsters will all see around 2,400 junk food adverts a year, every year from the ages of 2-18. That's just under 40,000 junk food ads through their childhood. It's hard to imagine that not having an impact.

In the UK, companies spend a vast amount of money on advertising junk food; it's been estimated by the British Medical Journal as 30 times the amount the Government spends on promoting healthy foods. Research by Cancer Research UK and Stirling University showed obese children remembered more junk food adverts on TV than healthy children.

Some countries are further ahead than others in terms of trying to control such advertising. Quebec in Canada has implemented a ban on junk food advertising on children's television, Norway has banned junk food advertising, France requires healthy messages as balance. There is a healthy debate in the UK, with 2018 law changes meaning no junk food advertising when Under 16's are the target audience of a programme. Many countries limit the placement and type of advertising aimed at children.

Back in the UK, KFC was censured in the UK for placing a Mars drinks advert too close to a school, while Kellogg's had their ads for Coco Pops

Granola banned by the Advertising Standards authority because of its links with the less healthy Coco Pops – though the power of the food industry was shown when Kellogg's successfully got that decision overturned.

Advertisers do not just target children's programmes; increasingly they target family programmes – which makes any legal limit harder to police. America's Got Talent is prominently sponsored by Dunkin' Donuts, and the UK's X Factor by Just Eat, the takeaway delivery app. The lack of restrictions on ads also applies to soaps, reality TV, and sports coverage.

Celebrity chef Jamie Oliver, who also launched a campaign to improve the nutritional quality of school dinners, believes there should be a 9pm watershed for junk food adverts.

"If kids are constantly being targeted with cheap, easily accessible, unhealthy junk food, just think how hard it must be to make better, healthier choices. We have to make it easier for children to make good decisions," explains his official website.

"These ads undermine any positive work we're doing in schools or at home to tackle the rise of childhood obesity. Currently, there's nothing in place to protect our kids from seeing these adverts – apart from literally covering their eyes! And that's where our #AdEnough campaign comes in…"

Any action in this direction would be welcome; anything short of the Quebec response of a total ban will have a limited effect. If parents see the adverts and children see some adverts, I fear the impact will still be significant. While bans are still worth doing, there should be a significant effort put into counter-messages.

Bad sports

Sports drinks and energy drinks have become hugely popular in recent years even though they are utterly unnecessary for anyone other than elite sports people and extremely hard trainers. For everyone else, they are a bit like taking vitamin tablets – a way of creating expensive urine!

Just as cigarettes contain all sorts of addictive elements which are not strictly necessary to create the nicotine hit, these energy drinks also contain addictive levels of sugar, in particular, and often caffeine as well.

There is a hidden danger in hooking in young people at an age when their bodies use much more energy. Even if they are thin youngsters, it is a bad and pointless habit. As they get older, their metabolisms will change and may not be able to cope. Those drinks add to the risks of careless obesity.

The UK Government is considering banning sales of energy drinks to Under 18's in England after evidence that two-thirds of children between the ages of 10-17 drink them. A quarter of 6-9 year-olds also consume the drinks. UK sales to children are 50% higher than for mainland Europe, for instance.

Some supermarkets are taking unilateral action, banning the sales of energy drinks to the Under 18s, which is a positive move. There are lifestyle questions in terms of younger people using such drinks to compensate for a lack of sleep because of the time spent on computer games or social media – but that is a whole new debate.

In the Punjab province of Pakistan, the authorities made drinks manufacturers drop the word 'energy' from their labels because it was scientifically misleading, which is another interesting approach.

Suffice it to say, there are plenty of parents and teachers who would welcome a ban on energy drinks to the Under 18s for behavioural reasons; a chance to kill two birds with one stone. Keeping children to water and squash would be one easy win in the fight against obesity.

There are some signs that obesity rates in children are beginning to slow down in the more advanced parts of the world (and even reverse) as our understanding has grown since the turn of the century. We understand the ramifications better and the importance more. Most parents are more aware than 15-20 years ago.

There are good examples to follow.

Taking action on action

As children get less freedom when outdoors (for safety reasons), so their activity levels outside school have dropped. There is a naturally safe environment where we can reverse that trend – and that is in school.

Elaine Wylie, the headteacher of St Ninian's primary school in Stirling in 2012, realised that her pupils were not particularly fit. When she sent them running around the school playing fields, they struggled. Afterwards, pupils and teacher decided to change their routines, and a daily group run around the playing fields was the result. It quickly extended to other classes and then the whole school.

Fitness levels improved, obesity dropped to low or non-existent, and a campaign for The Daily Mile was born. Sending children outside for a run or walk during lesson time is an idea which has been picked up by thousands of schools around the world. University of Stirling research proved the blindingly obvious – that children who did this were fitter, and had better body compositions, than children who didn't.

The Scottish Government 'promotes' the policy, but there has been a reluctance by politicians to push too hard. Firstly, they are held back by the belief that exercise is up to the individual; secondly, there is a reluctance to impose further red tape. They should just find a way of doing it! They should make it clear to all schools that this is an objective they should find their own way of achieving. It is not about target setting and measuring, just a clear objective for all schools.

There are two significant changes for children in terms of primary school, in particular. We all battle to drop our children off as close as we can to the front gate. At my children's primary school, that can literally mean a steady flow of parents stopping on the zebra crossing immediately outside the school to drop off their kids! If we all parked a few hundred yards away and walked, then that would be a start.

Secondly, primary school children often get taught in the same classroom all day, every day. Simply finding ways to move them around the school throughout the day should be a priority. Because we have an obsession with hard exercise a couple of times a week, we have forgotten about low-level activity. While I would personally love to see Physical Education as a daily subject in all primary schools, occasional organised PE is less of an answer than plenty of activity.

Ensuring children walk a mile a day should be a clear directive to all schools, part of an inspection report maybe, but not something that needs any off-putting red tape. No school should ever have to fill in forms saying they had fulfilled those terms; it is a simple question to the children when a school inspector calls, at most. If they only do a kilometre a day, then that's fine. Teachers want to do the right thing, so let's trust them.

Children can run or walk; it makes no difference. Some will see it as an athletic challenge, others as a chance to get out of lessons and chat for 15 minutes. It can be fun or challenging, or both. It is not a big deal; it need not involve changing into PE kit, it would just be something that happens as part of the daily routine.

The benefits are huge. Not only will there be a guaranteed level of activity every day in a safe environment, it will build up fitness, it will build up muscle development, all of which have a lasting impact on metabolism. Because such activity is routine and easy, it is likely to lead to more activity away from school. In many, it will trigger exercise hormones.

Lifestyles are less active as we are more concerned about the risks of being 'out and about.' It has led the Children's Commissioner for England, Anne Longfield, to warn about a "battery hen existence" for many kids; kids who spend their time indoors on computers and phones.

There is also a correlation between the number of fast food outlets around schools and the weight of nearby children. That is an area for town planners to take more seriously.

Of course, there are things we can do at home with our children, but we have moved towards occasional organised sport rather than letting them loose in the park for a couple of hours a day. I understand the changes and would not personally let young children go to the park on their own, (as I used to do when I was young) for obvious safety reasons. However, if we identify the issue, then we can do something to compensate.

One more small point about schools. Many clamp down on trainer-type shoes as going against uniform rules. Why? I understand rules on the colour of shoes, and branding, but what is wrong with shoes which make it easier for children to run and be active? We put an emphasis on smart uniforms; maybe we should look at school dress to promote active lifestyles?

However, when Telford Junior School in the Midlands of England tried to change the uniform to smart PE kit, they faced a revolt from some parents. The complaints ranged from the extra cost of school-branded hoodies, to making their kids look like chavvy drug dealers! One of the barriers to PE lessons is the time and effort to change clothes; this move was designed to be a way around that. Anything which encourages greater physical activity in school should be applauded.

If children are healthier and develop the muscles they need to walk and run at an early age, then those muscles will help burn calories and maintain the ease of exercise throughout their lives.

Anti antibiotics

We know the make-up of the bacteria in our gut has a significant impact on how our bodies cope with food and calories through our lives because of the microbiome.

Environments which are too sterile for young children can often be counter-productive in terms of the development of the anti-immune system. Indeed, the so-called Hygiene Hypothesis is credited by some with an increase in allergic reactions in the developed world that is not mirrored in less developed areas.

There has also been a new link with obesity in children if they have been given antibiotics before the age of two. Treatment for stomach acid may also have an effect, though the link is weaker.

This comes from an American military study[68] of more than 300,000 children up until the age of eight, who had received healthcare through the US military system.

The study found that roughly four out of every five children who became obese had been treated with antibiotics before the age of two. When other treatments, such as those for stomach acid, were taken into account, the figure of obese children who had not been through the treatments dropped to around one in 10. The theory is that these treatments may affect the balance of the stomach.

Trick or treat

The California Milk Processors Board calculated the average child's bucket on Halloween contains around 9,000 calories. You will be unsurprised to hear that this non-traditional trend was sparked by marketing from the candy industry in 1950's America, switching their attention from promoting Candy Day (which took place a couple of weeks later and which was, itself, a nakedly commercial invention back in 1916). However, the candy industry was pushing at an open door; small sweets were a popular gift for the traditional trick-or-treaters because of simplicity and ease.

We give children far more sugar at times like Halloween and Christmas than used to be the case. I buy a bucket load of sweets for the children who come knocking on our door at Halloween – anything else would be Scrooge-like (to mix up my holiday references).

I'm not sure we can put the genie back in the bottle.

If we are looking for an example of how to tackle the wider problems, there is a very simple one to follow in Amsterdam. They have found ways to reduce childhood obesity by 12% – a remarkable result in anyone's books.

The methodology is simple, with the starting point being as straightforward as having a coordinated response. They test children for weight and agility. They target overweight children with free exercise opportunities. A nurse looks at individual lifestyles to target specific issues rather than generalities. They also offer healthy eating advice, and they encourage people to cook their own food and include loads of vegetables. They target the poorer communities, which are often immigrant communities, with a particular emphasis on those buying and cooking the food. They have also targeted junk food advertising and sports sponsorship.

"We have managed to build a whole systems approach in Amsterdam," Karen den Hertog, Deputy Programme Manager, told the BBC.

"In the everyday life of children and their parents, we manage to get the healthy message across and help people have a healthier lifestyle. Once we decided what the message was, we were surprised by the enthusiasm from all our partners – youth workers, schools, teachers, doctors and nurses."

Amsterdam's budget for all this is around £5million. Maybe the fact they have recognised society can act, rather than blaming the individual, is a key to success.

Crucially, this shows that lower-income households can be targeted and can improve. They can be educated if you encourage the right family members. They may not be able to afford the perfect diet, but healthy food can be cheap and it is possible to improve diets within any budget. Not everyone has to eat avocado, salmon, and quinoa to improve their health.

The success of the scheme, since it started in 2012, is well known. The simplicity is clear to see. The effectiveness is clear to see. And still, it is not copied lock, stock, and barrel in many other places. People try to overcomplicate. People insist on clinging to 'eat less, exercise more,' rather than, 'provide information and offer opportunities.'

We need to educate children about healthy living. Maybe, once, it was parents and grandparents doing the teaching, but schools now have a role. It's not about some pompous lecture, which children generally ignore, and it should not be focused on weight. It should emphasise nutrition, the reasons for a balanced diet, and give them all the tools to cook for themselves in the healthiest possible way. My children have done cooking in school, but they have done cakes, cookies, pasties, and pizzas. Instead, it should be proper lessons on how to cook, plus education about the contents of microwave, oven-ready, and processed meals. How foods are farmed, processed, which fats are good and bad, the impact of storage versus fresh, what is in junk food that makes it bad – these are all areas perfectly suited for education. Lessons on food marketing techniques versus reality would not go amiss, either.

This should not be sermonising, but simply informing. Vegetarianism and veganism are growing trends among young people, thanks partly to social media. Children are interested in looking good. So simpler messages promoting healthy, non-gimmicky eating should be just as easy to push.

We need to create a revolution where we go back to cooking for ourselves, and the best chance is to start with the kids. In Amsterdam, they had success educating parents and carers, but of course the children of today will be the parents and carers of tomorrow. Again, if we can see a change in 5 or 10 percent, then that will have a significant impact for the rest of their lives. That is far more effective than trying to encourage them to diet.

Encouraging the next generation to stay active, avoid sugary drinks, and eat less processed food would probably be the biggest forward step we could make in reducing obesity in the long-term.

CHAPTER 15

The Future 4:
What We Can Do for Ourselves

"Healthy stuff is still healthy, it just doesn't make you thin."
Traci Mann, University of Minnesota

So, is there any hope? Is there any point in even trying to lose weight? We know it won't work in at least four out of five cases, so what's the point in trying?

To both those points, I would answer an emphatic YES! We have to try, but we have to re-assess our targets. We have to forget the messages and the methods of thin people who think their secret is something other than lucky genes, microbiome, or leptin efficiency. We have to make the best of what we have got, rather than chasing a fantasy.

The scientific research shows we can lose a significant amount of weight and keep it off by heeding the messages below. For some – particularly Lifestyle Fatties – that can mean achieving their aims. People who should not really have become overweight in the first place will find it easier to reverse. At the other end of the scales, we can still see some major improvements in quality of life.

We all have the target of getting thin and staying thin. All the weight loss award winners start and finish at different weights, but to win they must end up fully thin. Almost all the magazine articles about weight loss are about people who are thin, often going from fairly thin to very thin. We have all the thin experts telling other people how to be like them. In many cases, the judgement on whether we should follow advice is based on nothing more than the attractiveness of the person delivering it. That is even more the case with the advance of social media.

'Thin' is King. That is the expectation and the pressure, but it is an unlikely long-term result for many. We have to change our approach. Diets are out; life change is in. Willpower is out; self-analysis is in. Nothing is short-term, everything is about long-term plans – which will be more achievable if they allow for some short-term blips. Being thin would be nice, if it happens, but being healthier is much more achievable.

It's a message not all health professionals want you to know, as University of Alabama professor Tim Caulfield told CBC in 2014. "You go to these meetings and you talk to researchers, you get a sense there is almost a political correctness around it, that we don't want this message to get out there. You'll be in a room with very knowledgeable individuals, and everyone in the room will know what the data says and still the message doesn't seem to get out."

You're still fat, well done!

No-one has ever gone up to a friend or family member and said, "Well done; you look just as fat as last year!"

Why not? If you are one of the inch-a-year brigade, and you put a stop to that gradual growth, then that should be something to celebrate. An inch every two years would be an improvement and an achievement. Some praise would make you feel better and help stave off some of the negatives which fuel eating. The hair shirt attitude, and the criticism, are actually blocking the chances of making things better.

There is a strong link between depression and obesity. What has taken time to work out, is whether depression causes obesity or the other way around.

The largest study of its kind, carried out in the UK and Australia,[69] has found that the genetic variations likely to lead to obesity are also found in people likely to be depressed. This is based on half a million people between the ages of 37-73 registered in the UK Biobank. The link was stronger in women than in men. Researchers believe the link to be psychological, rather than biological; in other words, being fat is the cause of making us feel worse about ourselves.

That makes a lot of sense to me, but if we can change our thinking and our guilt about being fat, that may be a start to reducing the connection between obesity and depression. Of course, that is easier said than done, but we need to try to be positive about what we can achieve rather than worrying about what other people think. Hopefully, after reading this book and working some things out for yourself, you will know that you understand it so much better than the critics.

The biggest problem of putting on weight is the gradual increase over time. The second biggest problem is yo-yo weight going up and down. So why can we not celebrate slowing down or stopping that process? Why do we have to focus only on substantial weight loss, even though every study shows it is likely to be pointless in the long-run?

Maintaining the same level of weight would actually be good, especially for younger people, but reducing it by 5-10% should be achievable in many cases. 2012 research by the National Heart Forum in the US found that reducing average BMI by just 5% by 2030 would see millions of Americans spared from diseases.

There has been a move towards accepting who we are, as overweight people, rather than criticising. Body Positivity means loving who you are; Body Neutrality means acceptance. It is a welcome fightback against the criticism and verbal or typed vitriol aimed at higher profile overweight people. It reduces the obsession with weight loss and allows us to concentrate on other areas of health.

Target practice

To explain how we can achieve our new goals, I am going to start with golf. OK, a little different, but I am going to illustrate my point on how we should approach obesity by talking about the finishes to two Major golf championships.

The first relates to Scottish golfer Colin Montgomerie at the 2006 US Open at Winged Foot. Monty had, for years, been dubbed the best player never to win a Major (one of the big four golf tournaments each year). Then came the 2006 US Open – and it seemed as though his luck had changed as the breaks went his way.

Faced with a routine approach shot to the last green to win the title, he was forced to wait – and wait – for his playing partner to consult a referee. Doubts crept in. He would be inhuman if he did not have thoughts about what it would be like to win the US Open – the Major he had craved so desperately to round off his career. Montgomerie sliced his subsequent shot into trouble and consequently lost. In retrospect, he believes that if he had walked up to the ball and hit it without time to think, he would have found the green and won the title. Instead, after that lengthy delay, with all sorts of thoughts rushing through his mind, he hit one of the worst shots of his life.

Contrast that with South Africa's Louis Oosthuizen at The Open Championship at St Andrew's in 2010. He went into the final round with a comfortable lead, and it would have been easy to get ahead of himself, thinking about what it would be like to be a Major champion.

Oosthuizen had a little red dot marked on his glove. He looked down at that as he started his pre-shot routines and nothing else mattered, not whether it was the right shot to attempt, nor what it could mean; nothing apart from the red dot in front of him and his associated pre-shot routine. He cleared his mind and won.

All sports psychologists will tell you that if you concentrate on the long-term desire, then you are setting yourself up for failure. Instead, you concentrate on each step of the process which will get you there.

Concentrate on the training session at hand, or event, not the long-term wish to win Olympic gold. Focus on each round, not the eventual result; each shot, not the long-term goal; the next game... you get the idea. It is all about the process, not the end goal. It is about staying in the moment and doing your best every step of the way. If you do that, the long-term results will take care of themselves.

I think there are clear lessons for people trying to lose weight, or aiming to put on less weight. For most people, trying to be thin is like the golfer dreaming of winning rather than concentrating on the next shot. We need to completely re-assess our objectives as well as how we set about chasing them – and that does not just apply to us... this re-thinking has to apply to our support groups as well.

Rule makers, not rule takers

We know people who lose weight in the long-term are the exception, rather than the norm. The rest of us need to do the best that we can.

We need some ground rules to start off with.

Rule One. Being overweight is like any addiction. You are never cured; your genetics and hormones will never change (unless science takes a hand). It is a battle you will face every day of your life, but it is a battle you can win as long as the definition of victory is realistic. It is also a battle where you have to work out what is best for *you* in the feast or famine equation.

Which is why **Rule Two** is so important. Do not go on a diet, unless you have a specific reason for only wanting short-term weight loss

Rule Three. Weigh yourself every day. This is for information, not inspiration. The results are for your eyes only, not something you post on Facebook or declare at meetings. We are all different; there are millions of potential gene combinations affecting obesity. Weighing yourself every day will give the clearest idea of what works – or doesn't work – for you.

Rule Four. Cook for yourself, or enjoy someone else's home cooking, but either way, reduce the amount of fast food and packaged food that passes your lips. Rely on natural nutrition, and don't be swayed by marketing.

Rule Five. Forget salad. OK, this is a personal thing because of the number of people who have told me to eat more salad, and the number of phone-in comments I've heard, but it's a complete waste of time and resources.

Rule Six. Exercise, but this next sentence is really important. *I don't exercise because I think it will help me lose weight – I exercise because I know it won't!* That may sound odd, but I'll explain why it gives me more of a reason to exercise than the traditional messages, below.

Rule Seven. For anything else, refer to Rule One.

They are lessons I've learned the hard way. Like pretty much every overweight person in the world, my target when dieting or exercising has been to get thin. The failure to get thin is dispiriting, which in turn kickstarts our hunger hormones. Our new targets have to be in line with the growing body of science, not based on the prejudices of people with more fortunate genes.

The great thing is that realistic targets are more achievable, achievable targets are more motivating, more motivation helps you stick to your plans, all of which means the long-term results this way are better than setting some unrealistic aim.

Rule One

My name is Hamish, and I am an obese-aholic.

The bottom line is that all addictions, including over-eating, are a genetic and hormonal propensity which will never go away. As Cambridge University's Professor Sadaf Farooqi said after a new 2019 report,[70] "This research shows for the first time that healthy thin people are generally thin because they have a lower burden of genes that increase a person's chances of being overweight and not because they are morally superior, as some people like to suggest. It's easy to rush to judgment and criticise people for their weight, but the science shows that things are far more complex. We have far less control over our weight than we might wish to think."

We are what we are, but we have to try to make the best of the cards we have been given.

It is a long-term slog, every day of your life, with a few ups and plenty of downs. To succeed at all, you will go hungry for at least part of almost every day for the rest of your life; that is the reality. Not just a bit peckish, "you should show more control" sort of peckish… achingly, stomach-churningly, back-of-the-throat tingling hungry.

To change in the long-run, we have to go through every aspect of our lives, concentrating on habits rather than occasional treats or one-offs. This is nowhere near as simple as a short-term calorie-controlled diet, which takes no account of our hunger hormones.

Reducing our weight, or slowing down the gains, boils down to one question. What changes can *we live with* for the rest of our lives? There will be days when we slip back to old habits, without doubt, but not punishing ourselves is part of the process.

It means there is nothing too big or too small to look at, because tiny changes become big over a long period of time. We may not stick to these every day of our lives, but we are finding a new direction of travel. If we take a wrong turn here and there, then imagine the satnav calmly telling us the way back – "At the next opportunity take a U-turn" – rather than an irate passenger screaming and shouting, "Why did you do that, you stupid bleep bleep bleep bleeping bleep."

The starting point is what's known as empty calories. Of course, in reality, there is no such thing as empty calories because they still have an effect on our bodies; many create desire over a period of time. However, there are plenty of calories which do little to fill us up. Cutting those out, or reducing them as much as possible, is a good thing. Drinks are an obvious starting point; your body may crave them, but they do not fill us up.

The worst offenders are alcohol, concentrated fruit juices, milkshakes, sugary coffees, most commercially available drinks – even bottles of flavoured water have loads of sugar.

It might mean cutting out orange juice with breakfast or a regular glass of wine in the evening. It could mean cutting out energy drinks before or after activity. It could be cutting out a low calorie or zero calorie drink because they are stuffed full of unnatural sweeteners and trigger the body to absorb more calories from other foods.

Next up are snacks, especially if that means processed goodies such as most chocolates or biscuits. Why those? Because, in different ways, they are crammed full of extra sugars, trans fats, HFC, preservatives and the rest of the unnatural products our bodies find hardest to cope with. If you need any of these, then look for substitutes that still reduce those cravings. Homemade cake would be better than shop-made cookies, for example. Nuts are healthier than crisps or biscuits, though still high in calories and usually salty.

'Diet snacks' are generally as bad as any other kind. They may include some healthy ingredients they can boast about on the packet, but will often include unhealthy ones to bind them together and preserve them. Rarely will they be genuinely filling, so even if they are low calorie they will still be extra calories.

But here is another important part of my lifestyle-changing plan. If something is hard to give up, don't. Find ways of reducing it, because that will be more likely to stick over the long-term. Thin experts are forever telling us to give things up, because that is easy for them. My only principle is to find ways of making things better than they were before, better balanced and healthier. Try to find answers that are better, rather than perfect.

For example, there was one lady on the US TV programme The Weight of the Nation who had lost more than 100lbs and was keeping going from her starting point of over 400lbs, around 30 stone. One of her eating habits was a daily Kit Kat. Unfortunately, where she worked, she was surrounded by temptations. Her solution was not to give up Kit Kats altogether – that was not realistic for her – instead, she would break a Kit Kat in half, throw one half in the bin and then eat the other half.

The programme's researcher asked the question I did not need to ask. "Why do you throw half in the bin?" Why not keep it for the following day? The answer is that the other Kit Kat half would burn away at the lady's brain and would almost always get eaten on the same day. Throwing it in the bin got it out of harm's way.

Almost everyone going on a quick weight loss programme cuts something out of their diet, often carbohydrates, fats or sugars. We need all those things if we are going to be healthy for the rest of our lives. We also need all those things if we are to function at our best. We need those things if we are to lose fat rather than muscle, with the negative impact that has on our metabolic rate.

So, if you cannot give up a habit, try to make it better. If it is a nightly glass of wine, try to make sure it is rarely more than one glass. Is it possible to give up most Mondays? If it is, then how about Tuesdays too? The point is not to set yourself up to fail, because then you slip back into all your old habits. If you drink orange juice with breakfast, will water do instead? If you have two cans of cola – diet or non-diet, it doesn't really matter – then can you make it one? The point is to do something better than before – even if it is throwing half a Kit Kat in the bin.

We have made a start with drinks. The next stage is to look at breakfast to find out the healthiest way of filling yourself up. Can you replace cereal with porridge (made with water and oats, maybe add a dash of milk and fruit)? What about eggs instead of some chocolate-coated temptation? Can you cut out toast, or at least change from the most processed bread to something wholegrain?

Now we're on a roll. What about lunch? What do you eat in the office canteen; does it involve chips or are there other non-salad alternatives? Do you get a takeaway? What do we eat, where, and can we do it better (most days, if not every day)? What is practical for you to take to work for lunch? Look for healthy answers that fill you up, rather than low-calorie recommendations which leave you snacking later.

Now we're cooking with gas. How often is dinner a takeaway or something out of a packet or a jar? For example, a filling dish of pasta and sauce sounds healthy but is actually up there with the 'as bad as it gets' for calories and unnatural ingredients. How often can you cook for yourself with better ingredients and fewer additives? Make your own pasta sauce with chopped tomatoes, vegetables, herbs, and spices. Bulk the pasta out with added vegetables. If time is short, then can you make something at the weekend which will freeze or keep for a few days?

If you eat better main meals, do you snack less? Does a healthy evening meal cut out the midnight munchies? Try to eat better, not necessarily less. For example, if you find you can snack on fruit, then it will be fairly high-calorie, but those calories are shrouded in fibre, which helps the digestive system and also makes the sugars harder to ingest. Fruit doesn't impact my hunger much, but people are different.

It is all about trade-offs; whatever provides the healthiest, lowest calorie, *filling* solution. Satisfying your Inner Jolly Green Giant is the starting point for long-term success. If that means chocolate cake for breakfast, then so be it.

Regular meetings help people with other addictions; getting together with people suffering in the same way for mutual support. Many of the best counsellors have suffered from the same addiction, so they can offer realistic advice. Everyone sits around and says how hard it is, reinforcing the fact that it really is hard.

In contrast, weight loss meetings are led by thin people. To work for Weight Watchers, you have to be within 10lbs of your target weight; to work for Slimming World, you have to be 'close' to your target weight. Anyone who puts the weight back on loses their job, even though (to me) that would make them far more realistic group leaders. Instead of comparing stories about how hard it is, you are told how easy it is by people who mostly have no real understanding and who often provide messages which have failed time and time again over the long-term.

The branding change of Weight Watchers to WW, with a new emphasis on health rather than weight-loss, is an interesting step in the right direction. It was a reaction to people losing faith in diets and numbers in their schemes dropping. They added a million more members in 2017-18 after changing their emphasis away from weight towards well-being. It was also helped by brand ambassador and 10% owner Oprah Winfrey. The underlying message of concentrating on being healthy rather than weekly weighing sessions is very much in line with the advice in this book. So realistic meetings could help some people, but I do not like talking openly about such things; in common with many overweight people, I am shy. There are some things I don't want to admit to myself, never mind anyone else.

I hated Fat Class. Maybe it was the pain of being 'educated'; that I should do the things that make thin people thin. Maybe it was judging everything on intent rather than effectiveness; maybe it was the lecturing and hectoring. There were a couple of people of a similar view I could chat to on the way in and out, swapping tips and thoughts on what worked for us, and that was comfortably the only good bit.

Research shows we achieve more with good support, but I can't help feeling that, ultimately, we are on our own, with *our* support groups – for the rest of our lives. That is why it is so important that *our* support groups also buy into these messages, not the ones which have failed for 40 years.

Eating with other people helps limit our intake, but there has to be an all-round understanding that we will eat more to be satisfied. There is a danger of negative comments/nagging, but that is still better than eating on our own. Lack of satisfaction means eating more at other times; that's why we're fat.

So, whatever we decide to do has to be attainable for the rest of our lives. We will always try to improve our 'set' weight, but realistic targets are better than unrealistic ones.

Rule Two

The people peddling the 'diet' which worked for them are just different to you, genetically and hormonally. Their 'solution' has little or no relevance to you. The fact they are usually good looking is even less of a reason to follow them.

Short-term solutions are easy, no matter how hard, which is why they have proved popular. Diets are a thin person's answer to staying thin, no more. Unless you have a specific target you want to be temporarily thinner for – a wedding, a holiday, or an operation, for example – they are a waste of time and effort which would be better focused elsewhere.

There are three driving principles that have to apply. Anyone can recommend eating fewer calories, but for any changes to work long-term, they have to *stop you from feeling hungry for a reasonable amount of time*. If you are realistic about what you can stick to, for the rest of your life, then you will probably ignore most of the diet advice out there – but be better for it.

I know, for me, that weight which I'd lost was far, far easier to put back on. I know my body reacts differently depending on whether I have lost weight in the previous days, weeks, or months. It may have taken a couple of months to lose that weight, or longer, but I could put it back on in hours, as much as half a stone in one day. Boxers have been known to put on more than that in a day after getting down to their 'fighting weight.'

Perhaps the best way to explain this to thin people is to think of a time when you have been ill with a tummy bug, not eaten for a while, and lost weight – let's say half a stone for the sake of this argument. Under normal circumstances, it would take years for you to put on that amount of weight on top of your normal frame. How long does it take after being ill? Weeks? Days?

That would help to explain why the same diet starts really quickly in terms of weight loss and then slows down. It also explains why so many diets focus on quick results, because that is the comparatively easy bit and therefore commercially successful. When they go wrong, we blame ourselves, because of the early evidence the diet was working!

However – and this is really important to me – we should not think of a particular calorie intake as a daily test or target. I like thinking in terms of big numbers. Rather than thinking about how to stay below 2,000 calories a day, knowing there will be days when I fail to get anywhere near that, I would prefer to think of having somewhere between three quarters of a million and a little more than one million calories a year to play with, depending on size and activity levels. Falling off the wagon is not just inevitable, but at times it might be really useful, so thinking in terms of the big numbers allows for that. Falling off the wagon makes the Inner Jolly Green Giant relax for a while, in my experience, which may even be a good thing.

There is no point in doing anything for two weeks, three months, a year, or three years. You will kickstart your Inner Jolly Green Giant, your body will rebel, and the end result (five plus years down the road) is unlikely to be great and will probably be worse.

As part of that long-term view, do not use 'diet pills.' They vary from the useless to the dangerous. If scientists ever do bring out a pill which changes the microbiome to reduce weight, or changes our leptin receptiveness, or makes a genuine difference in some other way, then we will know about it. In the meantime, do not be conned by anyone claiming a magic solution.

Rule Three

I was struck by one of those programmes that followed slimming champions years afterwards and which found out they had nearly all put significant weight back on. These people who had weighed every ounce lost at one time had stopped weighing themselves as the numbers went up.

I did not weigh myself for around 30 years. I did not want to know; I did not feel I needed to know. I was fat; I was trying to do something about it – I didn't need to rub it in. All the messages about weighing yourself for inspiration and guidance always felt misguided to me. Unless you are thin, weighing yourself is depressing. Maybe I did not want to puncture my self-denial.

What changed? *I was weighed.* Then I had to weigh myself. If I wanted an operation to take away the crippling pain in my knee, then I had to break the habits of a lifetime.

What happened next was surprising, not least for me. Not because you watch the numbers going down and that inspires you to keep going. Not because you watch the numbers going up and that scares you into change.

But because weighing yourself every day gives you information. You know what you did the previous day, the previous week, the previous month. You learn what works and does not work with your body.

For instance, I learned that doing the same positive thing has diminishing returns. Just when you think you have cracked it, and the weight is coming off, you hit a brick wall even though you know you are doing the same actions. Weighing yourself every day can confirm how your body reacts differently, depending on what has gone before. I am so confident about the Inner Jolly Green Giant because I have witnessed the results on the scales every day – different results with the same intake, the same results with different intake – and that experience seems to tally with the anecdotes from overweight people and much of the scientific research.

It has given me the knowledge to back up, for myself at least, lots of things I thought before about how hard it is to lose weight, how wrong all the advice was, how hard it is to understand being fat unless you are fat.

I have evidence now about why much of what I did was always destined to fail, despite following the advice of someone-or-other who claimed to know what they were talking about. In the last few years, I have researched every area I can think of. Experimenting and weighing myself every day gives me real evidence about what works and does not work for me

Sometimes, I have bad days, and the weight goes up, but I can track it, and keep on top of it to a degree. Even if my weight is going up, there are no rude awakenings; I understand what is going on, it is all just part of the process.

I don't do it to punish myself, I don't write anything down, there are no targets, but it means I know where I am as well as the precise impact of certain behaviours and certain trends.

I know how hungry I felt the previous day and I know the impact any actions had on my weight. I am still searching for the Holy Grail of the fully satisfying day when you lose weight, but I am getting closer.

If you are serious about improving your life, then I believe weighing yourself every day, just for information, is central.

Rule Four

One Christmas, I was given a diet cookery book. I received it with a heavy sigh and with no expectations of any success – I have been given a lot of diet books in my time for some mysterious reason or other.

I tucked the book away and forgot about it. Then a few days later, going through a bag of Christmas presents that had not been the first things played with, I found it again. I flicked through it, saw it tallied with my own newly-changed thinking – and realised the recipes looked quite nice.

That book was The Hairy Dieters, the first of a series. The authors, Dave Myers and Simon King, are well-known as TV cooks 'The Hairy Bikers'. They are enthusiastic, with long hair, beards, and motorbikes, and travel around various places talking to local characters and finding out about the local food. They are down to earth, more likely to film in a backstreet takeaway than a Michelin-starred restaurant. They would fall into my definition of lifestyle fatties, rather than proper fatties. Neither is particularly large-framed and, naturally, a lifestyle of going around eating exotic foods is not conducive to weight loss.

Maybe that is hair-splitting – the bottom line is that they were overweight, took a look at themselves, and decided they had the culinary skills to do something about it.

That kickstarted me to cook for myself, largely with products which do not have lists of ingredients.

Aside from The Hairy Dieters, most cookbooks concentrate on making the nicest food, rather than the healthiest. However, there are plenty of places, particularly online, where you can find recipes with the aim of being healthy. You can also take pretty much any recipe and make it healthy by following some simple rules. Basically, bulk them out with loads of vegetables and some legumes (beans and lentils), to go with smaller amounts of protein and carbohydrate. Make sure you fill yourself up in the healthiest possible way. It helps that a diet with plenty of wholegrains, fibre, and balance will also be healthier.

I did not start eating better because I discovered willpower, but because the threshold dropped enough for me to be able to apply it. I have honestly shown much more willpower during periods of putting on weight than now, when I have lost some. I was obviously eating and drinking more than I should have then, but I was also turning my back on more things that I wanted.

It confirmed to me that the key to losing weight is finding food that is good for you that keeps the brain happy. The traditional emphasis of all the failed diets is the low-calorie food part; what we need to do is put our effort into finding the answer to keeping the brain happy.

I have very little doubt that the changes towards a healthier life will allow me to stay below my old weight – which was still slowly going in the wrong direction. Cooking for myself, cooking using reasonable ingredients, and ensuring plenty of vegetables on the plate – these allow me to 'partially' re-determine my set weight.

Other long-term eating plans are available, as the neutral BBC might say. The Paleo Diet (sometimes known as the caveman diet or Stone Age diet), for example, means eating the foods of our ancestors; more natural foods that our bodies evolved to cope with. I would applaud the move towards cooking proper ingredients, and avoiding modern processed food, but our ancient ancestors died pretty young, so there is a limit to how much the long-term effect of their diet was tested!

If you go to the British Nutrition Foundation, the Dietary Guidelines for Americans, Diabetes UK, the American Diabetes Association, or many others, then you actually get pretty boring advice. You can quibble over the realism of some of their recommended quantities, but the basic thrust of everyone is: plenty of natural products, plenty of fibre, and plenty of balance. Errrr, that's it.

But the one thing we cannot get away from is the basic maths of losing weight. Whatever we do has to fit within those pretty simple confines. There may be some leeway in terms of the exact content, but we have to put more good stuff (and less bad stuff) into our bodies over a long period of time.

Any time we fall off the wagon will count double or triple against us, so we have to find a wagon that can work for the foreseeable future. But it is not just simple maths; any methodology has to placate our inner Jolly Green Giant.

Cooking for ourselves should even extend to things like sauces to add flavour to our meals. 2018 Spanish research[71] presented to the American

Society of Clinical Oncology annual meeting in Chicago revealed how women using ready-made sauces – such as for curries and pasta – are almost three times more likely to develop breast cancer. Industrially produced breads and pies are also on the list of products linked to the disease.

Apart from anything else, eating better is likely to help more of us avoid depression – which in turn will help to reduce comfort eating. A 2018 study by researchers in Britain, Spain and Australia, published in the Molecular Psychiatry Journal, and based on 41 previous studies on links between diet and depression, showed poor diet is likely to cause depression, rather than just being associated with it. Foods containing lots of fats or sugars lead to inflammation all around the body.

Dr. Camille Lassale, of University College, London, the study's lead author, told The Guardian, "Chronic inflammation can affect mental health by transporting pro-inflammatory molecules into the brain, it can also affect the molecules – neurotransmitters – responsible for mood regulation." The report's authors even talk in terms of diet as a "psychiatric medicine."

Rule Five

We need an end to salad days. They are one of the biggest myths of the weight loss industry.

There are two types of salad. One, a genuine salad; full of lettuce, tomatoes, cucumber, and very few calories. Two, a fake salad, which has a bit of the above but plenty of pasta, mayonnaise, and calorie-filled dressings.

No-one thin believes me when I say this, but I can categorically state that when I eat a genuine salad, I am hungrier a couple of hours later than if I had eaten nothing at all.

It turns out there is science behind that belief; the same science that questions the validity of zero or low-calorie sodas. We know that you have to provide your body with nutrition of some sort, good or bad, for the internal 'House Full' signs to flash up. It turns out salads have an incredibly low nutritional value.

Dr. Charles Benbrook, formerly of Washington State, and Dr. Donald Davis, of the University of Texas, produced a 2011 report for The Organic Center: Identifying Smart Food Choices on the Path to Healthier Diets. The thrust of the research was eminently sensible, trying to find the most nutritious foods for the lowest number of calories. As part of that, they came up with a Nutritional Quality Index.

Salad scores appallingly badly on this list, largely because it is almost entirely water. Lettuce and cucumbers are 96% water, celery 95%, tomatoes 94%. Vegetables were slightly better, even though they are still around three quarters, or slightly more, water. Light salad scores comparatively highly by weight, but you would need to eat around 10 cups of lettuce, for instance, to start getting a nutritional value which stands up to a serving of vegetables.

So there really is little point in a genuine salad, before you consider the incredible quantities of food waste it causes – literally as our good intentions go to waste.

As a result, there is a small but significant lobby, led by the likes of The Washington Post and National Geographic, arguing that salad is one of the biggest wastes of the earth's resources in terms of land, water and fuel used to grow and transport it, along with the greenhouse gases in landfill from thrown away salad.

As food columnist, Tamar Haspel, wrote in The Washington Post, "There's one food, though, that has almost nothing going for it. It occupies precious crop acreage, requires fossil fuels to be shipped, refrigerated, around the world, and adds nothing but crunch to the plate. It's salad."

Suffice it to say, the next person who tells me to eat more salads will face an unexpected barrage!

But, if genuine salads are literally a waste of space, fake Salads are an even greater problem.

They fall under the 'health halo' which is more concerned about the attitude of a fat person than the effectiveness of behaviour. Tell someone you had a salad for lunch, and they will nod approvingly; never mind it may have been full of pasta and mayonnaise, and be well over a thousand calories.

The Santa Fe salad with tortilla, cheese, guacamole, or the Cobb salad with blue cheese, avocado, bacon, and chicken, to take just two examples, come in at well over 1,000 calories. Arguably the best of the crop, the Caesar Salad, is still just under 1,000 calories.

They can also include eye-watering quantities of salt, saturated fat, and preservatives. Just for comparison, a Big Mac contains 550 calories and less saturated fat than many salads.

Just as there are plenty of fats which get an undeservedly bad press, there are plenty of salads that get an undeservedly good press. Names can be deeply misleading.

A final story to illustrate the dangerous lure of such products. In our Fat Class, one member told the story about regular stays in a hotel and deciding to go out to buy a salad in a supermarket while others ate in the hotel restaurant. That sacrifice was praised as showing the right attitude even though the hotel meal was likely to be better balanced, more nutritious, and with fewer calories.

Rule Six

"Exercise is the single best thing you can do for yourself. It's way more important than dieting, and easier to do. Exercise works at so many levels—except one: your weight," wrote Robert H. Lustig in Fat Chance: Beating the Odds Against Sugar, Processed Food, Obesity, and Disease.

The problem with exercise is that it has been taken over by the exercise junkies – people who get a buzz and can't believe others don't.

It's time to reclaim exercise for all, but not for any of the reasons you will be told. If you are a few pounds overweight, then exercise may well be the key to getting the body you want. If you are much more overweight than that, then it may be the key to getting the body which will make your life better.

In other words, the focus is not on losing weight but developing our bodies to cope with being overweight. Once again, the target is being healthy rather than being thin.

In the UK, 87% of people do not use the gym. Of the remaining 13%, how many use the gym regularly?

There are two big reasons why fat people do not exercise more. 1. It's not very nice. 2. Being patronised, feeling uncomfortable, and out of place.

The problem with exercise is that it is driven by people who enjoy it, people who believe that last bit of effort driving through the pain barrier is vital. That is because, for them, it releases an endorphin and adrenaline rush which makes them feel good. They would not enjoy exercise as much without it, would not be driven in the same way, and they assume everyone is like that. But we are not.

I did a lot of sports training and lost count how often I was told sprinting the last few yards was the most important part. Of course, that's nonsense. The long part of the run, for example, was the important part. I was happy playing sport, but I hated training. I could get a rush from an event, a point, or a goal, but not from those last few yards – they just hurt and made me not want to do that again.

It's the same with jogging, swimming, exercise walking, and gym culture. It is all about exercising until it hurts.

We need to reclaim exercise; we need to make exercise pleasant so all we focus on the benefits. We do not need to do that last, unpleasant burst. Say, for example, you have used 300 calories cycling, finishing with a strong burst will use another 10. If the result of those last few calories is that you do not want to repeat the 300, then how is that a good idea?

I would urge you to join a gym, take up a sport, find something you enjoy which will involve you moving. It does not have to be hard; it could be bowls, golf, sailing – it could be some of the more active computer games. The more pleasant it is, the better. The more regular, the better. We do not need a weekly class to show willing; we need regular activities. This is too important to be a box-ticking exercise. This is about doing it often enough to change our bodies.

And don't push it. This is a change for the rest of your life, so stop short of the point that makes you want to stop.

Public Health England revealed in 2018 that aerobic exercise, the focus of so many fitness regimes, is only part of what you need to do. It is good for the heart, but we also need to develop our strength for more general wellbeing. That becomes especially important as we get older, but ties in with my own exercise regime which is focused on preparing my body to be able to carry my weight much more effectively. By building up my strength, as well as stamina, it turns out I am following Government advice.

Exercise will make your life more pleasant. Say you have knee problems… building up the muscles around the knee, the thighs, the gluteal muscles of the backside, and your back, will have a far greater impact than painkillers.

You do not need to make it unpleasant. Don't run, unless you enjoy that. Find somewhere nice to walk, rather than seeing walking as a chore. Amble pleasantly, rather than making it a route march. If you join a gym, then move around the equipment you like. Long, lung-bursting sessions on the treadmill are for the exercise junkies. Variety in exercise still uses plenty of overall calories, builds up more muscles, and means you are more likely to repeat. Choose exercise machines which are not weight bearing; you will feel a little like a normal person.

It will be a slow process, not a quick fix, but you will gradually feel better and better every day of your life.

Unfortunately, there is no way around being patronised at gyms, or while exercising out and about, until the attitudes of society change. When I talked about the joint pain of some exercises, I was told I needed to fight through that burn, and I would feel better. I had hoped that, eventually, this other person would get the message that pain meant pain – sharp, genuine, musculoskeletal pain – not aerobic discomfort. They didn't.

Then, a few months later, I was stopped on the sport centre's steps by a fellow gym goer who wanted to congratulate me on exercising and working at it, "although you have a lot to work on."

I smiled through gritted teeth and walked on.

There is a move to make gyms more attractive to the 87% who do not use them, rather than geared towards treating everyone like the 13%. It is a concept which started in Stockport back in 2009.

Life Leisure got rid of the mirrors, replaced pictures of fitness models with ordinary residents, installed anti-gravity treadmills so you do not feel your weight, cordoned off areas for anyone who is self-conscious, provided chairs for exercise, assigned obvious names for exercise classes such as 'Breathe Easy' or 'Breathe Hard' rather than just the latest fads.

"Gyms only appeal to people who already like gyms," CEO Malcolm McPhail told The Telegraph. "Our whole industry is about churn, people moving from place to place. We call it a gym for people who don't go to the gym."

The concept has been successful and has spread. Bigger gyms have taken on messages such as posters of ordinary people rather than fitness models.

It is an approach which has hope, but for me nothing beats walking in, keeping my head down, and doing my thing. I haven't lost weight, but my body feels much better. And, obviously, I have years and years of progress to go. I feel much healthier, so that ticks my box.

Two quick final points. By not flogging yourself in training, it will also be easier to avoid the idea of needing a 'reward' which cancels out the benefits. That can be a chocolate bar or drink other than water. Or it can be feeling you need a well-deserved rest, so the total level of activity drops. Secondly, as you build up, more muscles will have an impact on your metabolism, but don't expect major change to your weight.

A New Hope

OECD figures from 2017 showed that the obesity rates in the most developed countries are bad – but not without hope. Everyone focuses on the worst part of the figures – which usually involves the US and Mexico – but there are other areas worth learning from.

Countries like France, Italy, and Switzerland have stayed relatively stable since figures began in the 1990's. Spain had a slightly higher starting point, but obesity levels have dropped back down to the levels of the mid-1980's. UK levels have fluctuated since 2000 but stayed broadly stable. Canadian levels have only changed slightly since the early 1990's and are well below their neighbours in the US.

Clearly and understandably there is a focus on obesity in children, but levels have gone down for girls in the US, boys in France, and stayed pretty stable at a lower level for girls in France.

Obesity is not a one-size-fits-all problem. Some like to point towards the Mediterranean Diet as a potential route to follow. This was originally based on research which conveniently missed out various Mediterranean regions which would have complicated the argument, such as parts of France and Northern Italy. However, a visit to mid- and Southern European countries makes it extremely obvious why obesity levels are lower there. There is a focus on real food – vegetables, salad, even freshly made sweet food. There are more local food outlets and fewer multi-national brands. There is a strong, and surviving, cultural and social identity around food.

Part of the anti-obesity campaign is to play down the value of food and cooking. It seems areas where the opposite is the case are the most effective at countering the problem.

I will give one example which I believe sums up the differences. I spent time with an Italian who felt he was a few pounds overweight and was going on a diet to try and shift it. I asked what he would eat that evening, and he replied, "Pizza." Of course, our version of pizza for dinner would mean a takeaway or a prepared supermarket meal that was full of sugar, salt, preservatives, and calories – the opposite of going on a diet. His version was flour and water rolled into a base, topped with lots of fresh vegetables, a bit of meat, natural tomato sauce and mozzarella cheese. His version sounded great . . . and pretty healthy.

So, the picture is not as bad as some would have you believe. If the recommended BMI was changed to a more realistic level, so the figures became more representative of the problem, that would also help put things into better perspective.

And finally

Once we understand that obesity is nothing to do with diets and willpower, and everything to do with genetics, hormonal balance, microbiome, and modern eating habits, we can start tackling the problem effectively.

Once we stop concentrating on attitude and start looking at satisfaction, then we can educate people on realistic approaches.

Once we stop trying to punish fat people and start trying to understand them, then we can move forward constructively.

Once we point people towards the healthiest, nicest, filling foods, then we can make education effective.

Once we listen to fat people, rather than telling them to do things which all the evidence shows does not work, then we can find answers.

I do believe the current obesity crisis is made worse by changes in the way our society produces and encourages food provision, along with the way we live our lives. Clearly, it is a worldwide problem, rather than being the individual and separate fault of millions of fat people.

Governments and science hold the keys to the long-term answers.

However, whether it is 100 percent my fault, or 100 percent down to society, is pretty irrelevant. I have to live with it, and I have to find the best solution for me. You have to do the same for yourself.

Some help from governments and science would be good but, while waiting, I have to search for something. I cannot believe the bleakest picture; I cannot allow myself to. We have to find a way forward; we have to make improvements. I do not believe I will ever be properly thin, but I do believe I can be smaller than I was; I do believe I can stay around those levels and hopefully improve gradually over the long-term, staying smaller than I might have been.

The first thing is to try to make it easy to find a method that is not a punishment. Once we change our target towards living a healthier life, we can improve our situation. A lot of the illness and disease associated with obesity has plenty of evidence linking them to lifestyle. A change of emphasis could be empowering.

The old-fashioned plate of food would be roughly one-third meat or fish, one-third carbohydrate, and one-third vegetables. You can tweak the numbers around the edges, throwing in some legumes as well, but that still seems a pretty good approach. It is an approach I had gone away from when I used to follow a lot of diet advice.

Diets bombard you with so many messages; they frighten you off so many things. You take – and sometimes twist – the parts that can work for you. It gets complicated as you try to balance what you are told to do, and what you can do.

Balance is vital in your diet; so that rules out more of the long-term gimmicks. Our bodies have developed thanks to a wide range of proteins, carbohydrates, vitamins, fats, sugars, and the rest. If we cut out one form of food, which historically our bodies have needed, then we either need deep knowledge to make sure we replace that source of energy, or there is a good chance our health will suffer in the long run.

That negative impact could be decades later depending on what we cut out and for how long.

A Stanford University study, published in 2018, put a group on a low carbohydrate diet up against a group on a low fats diet for a year. Both groups were urged not to count the calories, but to concentrate on the types of nutrient-dense, whole food they were eating. Both groups were encouraged to maximise vegetables and cut back on the amount of added sugars, trans fats, refined grains, and processed food they ate. They were also encouraged to prepare food at home as much as possible. Both groups lost a little less than a stone per person on average over the 12 months.

Two very different diets, very similar results, so it seems the food quality was the key factor in gradual weight loss: unpackaged and prepared at home. The approach mattered more than the details of the diet.

As California-based health author and practitioner, Dr. Chris Kresser, an advocate of the Paleo Diet, explained, "When the subjects focused on real, whole foods and cut refined grains, sugars, and processed foods out of their diet, they lost significant weight, without having to count calories or restrict energy intake. However, this was based on averages, and does not mean that an individual might not respond better to a low-carb or low-fat diet."

Feeling satisfied is the most important thing; stopping the cravings building up, combatting the mid-afternoon snacking; and knocking the midnight bingeing on the head by eating better main meals.

It gets harder over time. The body's natural hormones kick back in, and some of the old habits are hard to break. I can completely see why any study of fewer than five years is worthless. It is around five years since I committed to all the research for this book and started experimenting with what I found. All the stuff written and spoken about the 'motivation' of losing weight is claptrap for me. The reality is that losing weight just makes it harder and harder to keep it off.

Once again, I would urge you to be realistic, and not to worry about perfect solutions but to find something better. It does not have to be unpleasant. In terms of food, it can be re-assessing what you eat rather than how much. In terms of exercise, it can be the old cliché of walking up the stairs at work rather than taking the lift; it could be getting a dog to go for more regular walks. It just takes a little bit of thought to find something that would fit into your life.

I am not trying to tell anyone what to do; I am in no position to prescribe solutions. The one thing I can do is offer ideas that have worked for me from the perspective of a fat person.

It won't get me on the cover of Slimming World, and no-one has been knocking on my door asking me to tell my 'dramatic weight loss story.' No-one has asked for me to be pictured holding out my old clothes to show how much weight I've lost. But I am happy I can be healthier for the rest of my life. There are no target weights or timescales. I'm not inspired or motivated, and I'm not working at it.

I think it is obvious to try to be the tortoise rather than the hare – and the worldwide figures seem to back up that approach.

One piece of good advice I was given at Fat Class was to eat as many foods as possible that do not come with a number of calories on them. If they are natural and unprocessed, then they have no labels for added content.

One of the few facts about the obesity debate is that, on average, the poorer are more likely to be obese than the wealthy. Of course, one of the central differences according to wealth will be the quality of food you can afford.

For all those people who have lost weight and kept the weight off, well done; whatever you did has obviously worked whether it was a crash diet followed by lifestyle change or an exercise regime – or both. There are plenty of Lifestyle Fatties who can achieve dramatic results.

For the massive majority who have found that diets do not work over five years or more, I honestly believe we need a new way of thinking – slow and steady lifestyle changes are the way forward. However, the overwhelming message would be that losing weight is extremely hard.

This is not a book by a good-looking person telling you how to copy them. Socrates said, "I cannot teach anybody anything. I can only make them think." Instead, use the information in this book to take time to understand what you can change, ignoring much of the advice out there.

As Narnia author, CS Lewis, put it, "We cannot go back and change the beginning. But we can start where we are and change the ending."

Find a way of eating home-cooking; if it means more regular, smaller shopping trips then that is no bad thing either. Do try to source better quality food – more local supply chains can mean it need not be more expensive.

Don't be fooled by the marketing. Foods that tell us they're healthy are nowhere near as healthy as natural foods that don't tell us anything. Distrust the food industry; the less you can use their processed products the better.

Like the top sportsmen and women, try to eat well-produced, natural food as much as possible – as much as budgets allow. Focus on the process of eating more healthily, not the end result of losing weight.

Weigh yourself every day, but only for information.

Look closely at what you drink; the easiest way of reducing calories without upsetting your Inner Jolly Green Giant.

Remember, this is something you have to do every day – or most days – for the rest of your life. Be realistic about what you can and cannot do.

In all probability, that will not mean becoming thin for ever more. It will involve a daily battle against the forces within us. But it can mean being healthier, happier, and better placed to cope with our lives.

Good luck. You can make a difference for yourself and others, just concentrate on the red spot rather than the end goal.

Welsh poet Dylan Thomas was talking about the death of his father in the poem Do Not Go Gentle into that Good Night. However, the final two lines also sum up my views on how we must fight that daily battle against modern food trends and obesity.

Do not go gentle into that good night,
Rage, rage against the dying of the light.

REFERENCES

[1] Trends in adult body-mass index in 200 countries from 1975 to 2014: a pooled analysis of 1698 population-based measurement studies with 19.2 million participants. The Lancet, 2-8 April 2016, Vol.387(10026), pp.1377-1396

[2] Led by Professor Andrew Hill from the Leeds Institute of Health Sciences. The research investigated young children's ratings of, and choices between, story characters drawn as overweight, normal weight, or disabled. The results of the study were presented at the European Congress on Obesity (ECO) in Liverpool.

[3] Centre for Creative Leadership research carried out after they spotted a trend concerning 750 peer reviewed managers in their leadership programmes.

[4] Is Obesity Stigmatizing? Body Weight, Perceived Discrimination, and Psychological Well-Being in the United States. Carr, Deborah ; Friedman, Michael A. Journal of Health and Social Behavior, September 2005, Vol.46(3), pp.244-259

[5] The relationship between body weight and perceived weight-related employment discrimination: The role of sex and race. Roehling, Mark V. ; Roehling, Patricia V. ; Pichler, Shaun. Journal of Vocational Behavior, 2007, Vol.71(2), pp.300-318

[6] *The Impact of Obesity on Wages. Cawley, John. The Journal of Human Resources, 1 April 2004, Vol.39(2), pp.451-474*

[7] *Weight Discrimination: A Multidisciplinary Analysis. Maranto, Cheryl ; Stenoien, Ann. Employee Responsibilities and Rights Journal, 2000, Vol.12(1), pp.9-24*

[8] *Does Body Weight affect Wages? Evidence from Europe. Brunello, Giorgio ; D'Hombres, Beatrice. IDEAS Working Paper Series from RePEc, 2006*

[9] *Investigating the Validity of Stereotypes About Overweight Employees: The Relationship Between Body Weight and Normal Personality Traits. Roehling, Mark V ; Roehling, Patricia V ; Odland, L Maureen. Group & Organization Management, August 2008, Vol.33(4), pp.392-424*

[10] Perhaps the most comprehensive is The Stigma of Obesity: A Review and Update. Puhl, Rebecca M. ; Heuer, Chelsea A.

[11] Men's preferences in romantic partners: obesity vs addiction. Sitton S1, Blanchard S. Psychol Rep. 1995 Dec;77(3 Pt 2):1185-6.

[12] Feeding Releases Endogenous Opioids in Humans. Tuulari, Jetro J ; Tuominen, Lauri ; de Boer, Femke E ; Hirvonen, Jussi ; Helin, Semi ; Nuutila, Pirjo ; Nummenmaa, Lauri. The Journal of neuroscience: the official journal of the Society for Neuroscience, August 23, 2017, Vol.37(34), pp.8284-8291

[13] A series of surveys conducted at the University of Chicago by the American Society for Metabolic and Bariatric Surgery (ASMBS) and NORC, funded by ASMBS and used AmeriSpeak®.

[14] Ego Depletion: Is the Active Self a Limited Resource? Baumeister, Roy F. ; Bratslavsky, Ellen ; Muraven, Mark ; Tice, Dianne M. Journal of Personality and Social Psychology, 1998, Vol.74(5), pp.1252-1265

[15] The Unbearable Automaticity of Being. Bargh, John A. ; Chartrand, Tanya L. American Psychologist, 1999, Vol.54(7), pp.462-479

[16] Medicare's Search for Effective Obesity Treatments. Mann, Traci ; Tomiyama, A. Janet ; Westling, Erika ; Lew, Ann-Marie ; Samuels, Barbra ; Chatman, Jason. American Psychologist, 2007, Vol.62(3), pp.220-233

[17] Weight-loss maintenance 1, 2 and 5 years after successful completion of a weight-loss programme. Lowe, Michael R ; Kral, Tanja V. E ; Miller-kovach, Karen. British Journal of Nutrition, 2008, Vol.99(4), pp.925-930

[18] Atkins and other low-carbohydrate diets: Hoax or an effective tool for weight loss? Astrup, P.A. ; Meinert Larsen, D.T. ; Harper, A. Lancet, 4 September 2004, Vol.364(9437), pp.897-899

and

A life-threatening complication of Atkins diet. Chen, Tsuh-Yin ; Smith, William ; Rosenstock, Jordan L ; Lessnau, Klaus-Dieter. The Lancet, 2006, Vol.367(9514), pp.958-958

[19] Short-term feeding of a ketogenic diet induces more severe hepatic insulin resistance than an obesogenic high-fat diet. Grandl, Gerald ; Straub, Leon ; Rudigier, Carla ; Arnold, Myrtha ; Wueest, Stephan ; Konrad, Daniel ; Wolfrum, Christian. Journal of Physiology, October 2018, Vol.596(19), pp.4597-4609

[20] Effect of Low-Fat vs Low-Carbohydrate Diet on 12-Month Weight Loss in Overweight Adults and the Association With Genotype Pattern or Insulin Secretion: The DIETFITS Randomized Clinical Trial. Gardner, Christopher D ; Trepanowski, John F ; Del Gobbo, Liana C ; Hauser, Michelle E ; Rigdon, Joseph ; Ioannidis, John P A ; Desai, Manisha ; King, Abby C. JAMA, 20 February 2018, Vol.319(7), pp.667-679

[21] Dietary carbohydrate intake and mortality: a prospective cohort study and meta-analysis. Seidelmann, Sara B ; Claggett, Brian ; Cheng, Susan ; Henglin, Mir ; Shah, Amil ; Steffen, Lyn M ; Folsom, Aaron R ; Rimm, Eric B ; Willett, Walter C ; Solomon, Scott D. The Lancet Public Health, September 2018, Vol.3(9), pp.e419-e428

[22] Effects of Different Doses of Physical Activity on Cardiorespiratory Fitness Among Sedentaryk, Overweight or Obese Postmenopausal Women With Elevated Blood Pressure: A Randomized Controlled Trial. Church, Timothy ; Earnest, Conrad ; Skinner, James ; Blair, Steven. JAMA, May 16, 2007, Vol.297(19), pp.2081-91

[23] State of Obesity: Better Policies for a Healthier America. Trust for America's Health & Robert Wood Johnson Foundation. https://stateofobesity.org/wp-content/uploads/2018/09/stateofobesity2018.pdf

[24] Effect of Short-term Exercise on Appetite, Energy Intake and Energy-regulating Hormones. Ebrahimi, Mohsen ; Rahmani- Nia, Farhad ; Damirchi, Arsalan ; Mirzaie, Bahman ; Asghar Pur, Sepide. Iranian Journal of Basic Medical Sciences, 2013, Vol.16(7), p.829-834

[25] Obesity Epidemiology: From Aetiology to Public Health. Crawford, D. ; Jeffery, R.W. ; Ball, K. ; Brug, J.

[26] Trends in physical activity, sedentary behavior, diet, and BMI among US adolescents, 2001-2009. Iannotti, Ronald J ; Wang, Jing. Pediatrics, October 2013, Vol.132(4), pp.606-614

[27] Evidence for a strong genetic influence on childhood adiposity despite the force of the obesogenic environment. Wardle, Jane ; Carnell, Susan ; Haworth, Claire ; Plomin, Robert. The American Journal of Clinical Nutrition, Feb 1, 2008, Vol.87(2), p.398

[28] He Was No Coward, The Harry Farr Story. Janet Booth and James White

[29] Eating as an automatic behavior. Cohen, Deborah ; Farley, Thomas A. Preventing chronic disease, Vol.5(1), p.A23

[30] Metabolic rates, climate and macroevolution: a case study using Neogene molluscs. Strotz, Luke C. ; Saupe, Erin E. ; Kimmig, Julien ; Lieberman, Bruce S. Proceedings of the Royal Society B: Biological Sciences, 08/29/2018, Vol.285(1885), p.20181292

[31] Sugar industry sponsorship of germ-free rodent studies linking sucrose to hyperlipidemia and cancer: An historical analysis of internal documents. Kearns, Cristin ; Apollonio, Dorie ; Glantz, Stanton. PLoS Biology, Nov 2017, Vol.15(11)

[32] Obesity Epidemiology: From Aetiology to Public Health. Crawford, D. ; Jeffery, R.W. ; Ball, K. ; Brug, J.

[33] Effects of Food Form and Timing of Ingestion on Appetite and Energy Intake in Lean Young Adults and in Young Adults with Obesity. Mattes, Richard D. ; Campbell, Wayne W. Journal of the American Dietetic Association, 2009, Vol.109(3), pp.430-437

and

Liquid versus solid carbohydrate: effects on food intake and body weight. Dimeglio D.P. ; Mattes R.D. International Journal of Obesity, 2000, Vol.24(6), p.794

[34] Consuming fructose-sweetened, not glucose-sweetened, beverages increases visceral adiposity and lipids and decreases insulin sensitivity in overweight/obese humans. Stanhope, Kimber L ; Schwarz, Jean Marc ; Keim, Nancy L ; Griffen, Steven C ; Bremer, Andrew A ; Graham, James L ; Hatcher, Bonnie ; Cox, Chad L ; Dyachenko, Artem ; Zhang, Wei ; Mcgahan, John P ; Seibert, Anthony ; Krauss, Ronald M ; Chiu, Sally ; Schaefer, Ernst J ; Ai, Masumi ; Otokozawa, Seiko ; Nakajima, Katsuyuki ; Nakano, Takamitsu ; Beysen, Carine ;

Hellerstein, Marc K ; Berglund, Lars ; Havel, Peter J. The Journal of clinical investigation, May 2009, Vol.119(5), pp.1322-1334

[35] Fructose as a key player in the development of fatty liver disease. Basaranoglu, Metin ; Basaranoglu, Gokcen ; Sabuncu, Tevfik ; Sentürk, Hakan. World journal of gastroenterology, Vol.19(8), pp.1166-1172

[36] A dose-response study of consuming high-fructose corn syrup-sweetened beverages on lipid/lipoprotein risk factors for cardiovascular disease in young adults. Stanhope, Kimber L ; Medici, Valentina ; Bremer, Andrew A ; Lee, Vivien ; Lam, Hazel D ; Nunez, Marinelle V ; Chen, Guoxia X ; Keim, Nancy L ; Havel, Peter J. The American journal of clinical nutrition, June 2015, Vol.101(6), pp.1144-54

[37] A dose-response study of consuming high-fructose corn syrup-sweetened beverages on lipid/lipoprotein risk factors for cardiovascular disease in young adults. Stanhope, Kimber L ; Medici, Valentina ; Bremer, Andrew A ; Lee, Vivien ; Lam, Hazel D ; Nunez, Marinelle V ; Chen, Guoxia X ; Keim, Nancy L ; Havel, Peter J. The American journal of clinical nutrition, June 2015, Vol.101(6), pp.1144-54

[38] Intake of sugar-sweetened beverages and weight gain: a systematic review. Malik, Vasanti S ; Schulze, Matthias B ; Hu, Frank B. The American journal of clinical nutrition, Vol.84(2), pp.274-288

[39] Relationship of soft drink consumption to global overweight, obesity, and diabetes: a cross-national analysis of 75 countries. Basu, Sanjay ; Mckee, Martin ; Galea, Gauden ; Stuckler, David. American journal of public health, November 2013, Vol.103(11), pp.2071-2077

[40] Diet-beverage consumption and caloric intake among US adults, overall and by body weight. Bleich, Sara N ; Wolfson, Julia A ; Vine, Seanna ; Wang, Y Claire. American journal of public health, March 2014, Vol.104(3), pp.e72-e78

[41] The effect of musical style on restaurant customers' spending. North, Adrian ; Shilcock, Amber ; Hargreaves, David. Environment and Behavior, Sep 2003, Vol.35(5), pp.712-718

[42] Perceived weight discrimination in England: a population-based study of adults aged 50 and older. S E Jackson ; A Steptoe ; R J Beeken ; H Croker ; J Wardle. International Journal of Obesity, 2014

[43] The ironic effects of weight stigma. Major, Brenda ; Hunger, Jeffrey M. ; Bunyan, Debra P. ; Miller, Carol T. Journal of Experimental Social Psychology, March 2014, Vol.51, pp.74-80

[44] Dr Sharma's Obesity Notes, Do Shame And Blame Tactics Make The Obesity Problem Worse? December, 2013. http://www.drsharma.ca/do-shame-and-blame-tactics-make-the-obesity-problem-worse

[45] Circulating Biomarkers of Dairy Fat and Risk of Incident Diabetes Mellitus Among Men and Women in the United States in Two Large Prospective Cohorts. Yakoob, Y., Mohammad ; Shi, C., Peilin ; Willett, M., Walter ; Rexrode, John, Kathryn ; Campos, B., Hannia ; Orav, B., E. ; Hu, B., Frank ; Mozaffarian, B., Dariush. Circulation, 2016, Vol.133(17), p.1645-1654

[46] The relationship between high-fat dairy consumption and obesity, cardiovascular, and metabolic disease. Kratz, Mario ; Baars, Ton ; Guyenet, Stephan. European Journal of Nutrition, 2013, Vol.52(1), pp.1-24

[47] Longitudinal evaluation of milk type consumed and weight status in pre-schoolers. Scharf, Rebecca J ; Demmer, Ryan T ; Deboer, Mark D. Archives of Disease in Childhood, 18 May 2013, Vol.98(5), p.335

[48] Meal timing and composition influence ghrelin levels, appetite scores and weight loss maintenance in overweight and obese adults. Jakubowicz, Daniela ; Froy, Oren ; Wainstein, Julio ; Boaz, Mona. Steroids, 10 March 2012, Vol.77(4), pp.323-331

[49] Chocolate consumption and risk of stroke: A prospective cohort of men and meta-analysis. Larsson, C., Susanna ; Virtamo, C., Jarmo ; Wolk, C., Alicja. Neurology, 2012, Vol.79(12), p.1223-1229

[50] Change in Body Mass Index Associated With Lowest Mortality in Denmark, 1976-2013. Afzal, Shoaib ; Tybjærg-Hansen, Anne ; Jensen, Gorm B ; Nordestgaard, Børge G. JAMA, 10 May 2016, Vol.315(18), pp.1989-96

[51] Lifestyle intervention: from cost savings to value for money. Rappange, David R ; Brouwer, Werner B. F ; Rutten, Frans F. H ; Van Baal, Pieter H. M. Journal of Public Health, 2010, Vol. 32(3), pp.440-447

[52] Worldwide trends in diabetes since 1980: a pooled analysis of 751 population-based studies with 4·4 million participants. Ncd Risk Factor Collaboration (Ncd-Risc); The Lancet, 9-15 April 2016, Vol.387(10027), pp.1513-1530

[53] Obesity. Published online at OurWorldInData.org. Hannah Ritchie and Max Roser (2018). https://ourworldindata.org/obesity

[54] Regulatory variants at KLF14 influence type 2 diabetes risk via a female-specific effect on adipocyte size and body composition. Small, Kerrin S ; Todorčević, Marijana ; Civelek, Mete ; El-Sayed Moustafa, Julia S ; Wang, Xiao ; Simon, Michelle M ; Fernandez-Tajes, Juan ; Mahajan, Anubha ; Horikoshi, Momoko ; Hugill, Alison ; Glastonbury, Craig A ; Quaye, Lydia ; Neville, Matt J ; Sethi, Siddharth ; Yon, Marianne ; Pan, Calvin ; Che, Nam ; Viñuela, Ana ; Tsai, Pei-Chien ; Nag, Abhishek ; Buil, Alfonso ; Thorleifsson, Gudmar ; Raghavan, Avanthi ; Ding, Qiurong ; Morris, Andrew P ; Bell, Jordana T ; Thorsteinsdottir, Unnur ; Stefansson, Kari ; Laakso, Markku ; Dahlman, Ingrid ; Arner, Peter ; Gloyn, Anna L ; Musunuru, Kiran ; Lusis, Aldons J ; Cox, Roger D ; Karpe, Fredrik ; Mccarthy, Mark I. Nature genetics, April 2018, Vol.50(4), pp.572-580

[55] Quantity and Quality of Sleep and Incidence of Type 2 Diabetes. Cappuccio, Francesco ; D'Elia, Lanfranco ; Strazzullo, Pasquale ; Miller, Michelle. Diabetes Care, Feb 2010, Vol.33(2), pp.414-420

[56] The 2016 global and national burden of diabetes mellitus attributable to PM2·5 air pollution. Bowe, Benjamin ; Xie, Yan ; Li, Tingting ; Yan, Yan ; Xian, Hong ; Al-Aly, Ziyad. The Lancet Planetary Health, July 2018, Vol.2(7), pp.e301-e312

[57] Mortality trends in patients with and without diabetes in Ontario, Canada and the UK from 1996 to 2009: a population-based study. Lind, M. ; Garcia-Rodriguez, L. ; Booth, G. ; Cea-Soriano, L. ; Shah, B. ; Ekeroth, G. ; Lipscombe, L. Diabetologia, 2013, Vol.56(12), pp.2601-2608

[58] Associations of fats and carbohydrate intake with cardiovascular disease and mortality in 18 countries from five continents (PURE): a prospective cohort study. Dehghan, Mahshid ; Mente, Andrew ; Zhang, Xiaohe ; Swaminathan, Sumathi ; Li, Wei ; Mohan, Viswanathan ; Iqbal, Romaina ; Kumar, Rajesh ; Wentzel-Viljoen, Edelweiss ; Rosengren, Annika ; Amma, Leela Itty ; Avezum, Alvaro ; Chifamba, Jephat ; Diaz, Rafael ; Khatib, Rasha ; Lear, Scott ; Lopez-Jaramillo, Patricio ; Liu, Xiaoyun ; Gupta, Rajeev ; Mohammadifard, Noushin ; Gao, Nan ; Oguz, Aytekin ; Ramli, Anis Safura ; Seron, Pamela ; Sun, Yi ; Szuba, Andrzej ; Tsolekile, Lungiswa ; Wielgosz, Andreas ; Yusuf, Rita ; Hussein Yusufali, Afzal ; Teo, Koon K ; Rangarajan, Sumathy ; Dagenais, Gilles ; Bangdiwala, Shrikant I ; Islam, Shofiqul ; Anand, Sonia S ; Yusuf, Salim. The Lancet, 4-10 November 2017, Vol.390(10107), pp.2050-2062

[59] Reversing Type 2 Diabetes, Professor Roy Taylor, Newcastle University, June 2018.

[60] Chocolate intake is associated with better cognitive function: The Maine-Syracuse Longitudinal Study. Crichton, Georgina E. ; Elias, Merrill F. ; Alkerwi, Ala'a. Appetite, 1 May 2016, Vol.100, pp.126-132

[61] Making China safe for Coke: how Coca-Cola shaped obesity science and policy in China. Greenhalgh, Susan. BMJ: British Medical Journal (Online), Jan 9, 2019, Vol.364

[62] Sugar reduction and wider reformulation: report on progress towards the first 5% reduction and next steps, Public Health England. https://assets.publishing.service.gov.uk/government/uploads/system/uploads/attachment_data/file/709008/Sugar_reduction_progress_report.pdf

[63] Nutritional labelling for healthier food or non-alcoholic drink purchasing and consumption. Crockett, Rachel A ; King, Sarah E ; Marteau, Theresa M ; Prevost, A T ; Bignardi, Giacomo ; Roberts, Nia W ; Stubbs, Brendon ; Hollands, Gareth J ; Jebb, Susan A. Cochrane Database of Systematic Reviews, 02/27/2018

[64] Nutrition-Labeling Regulation Impacts on Restaurant Environments. Saelens, Brian E. ; Chan, Nadine L. ; Krieger, James ; Nelson, Young ; Boles, Myde ; Colburn, Trina A. ; Glanz, Karen ; Ta, Myduc L. ; Bruemmer, Barbara. American Journal of Preventive Medicine, November 2012, Vol.43(5), pp.505-511

[65] Connection Between BMI-Related Plasma Metabolite Profile and Gut Microbiota. Ottosson, M, Filip ; Brunkwall, M, Louise ; Ericson, M, Ulrika ; Nilsson, M, Peter ; Almgren, M, Peter ; Fernandez, M, Céline ; Melander, M, Olle ; Orho-Melander, M, Marju. The Journal of Clinical Endocrinology & Metabolism, 2018, Vol.103(4), p.1491-1501

[66] Why are poorer children at higher risk of obesity and overweight? A UK cohort study. Goisis, Alice ; Sacker, Amanda ; Kelly, Yvonne. The European Journal of Public Health, 2016, Vol. 26(1), pp.7-13

[67] Childhood Obesity Facts. CDC Healthy Schools. 2017. https://www.cdc.gov/healthyschools/obesity/facts.htm

[68] Antibiotic and acid-suppression medications during early childhood are associated with obesity. Stark, Christopher M ; Susi, Apryl ; Emerick, Jill ; Nylund, Cade M. Gut, 30 January 2019, Vol.68(1), p.62

[69] Using genetics to understand the causal influence of higher BMI on depression. Tyrrell, Jessica ; Mulugeta, Anwar ; Wood, Andrew R ; Zhou, Ang ; Beaumont, Robin N ; Tuke, Marcus A ; Jones, Samuel E ; Ruth, Katherine S ; Yaghootkar, Hanieh ; Sharp, Seth ; Thompson, William D ; Ji, Yingjie ; Harrison, Jamie ; Freathy, Rachel M ; Murray, Anna ; Weedon, Michael N ; Lewis, Cathryn ; Frayling, Timothy M ; Hyppönen, Elina. International journal of epidemiology, November 13, 2018

[70] Genetic architecture of human thinness compared to severe obesity. Riveros-McKay F, Mistry V, Bounds R, Hendricks A, Keogh JM, Thomas H, et al. (2019) PLoS Genet 15(1): e1007603. https://doi.org/10.1371/journal.pgen.1007603

OTHER BOOKS FROM BENNION KEARNY

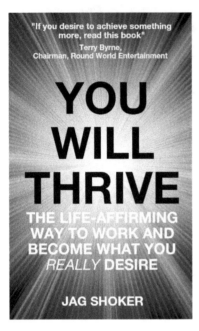

You Will Thrive: The Life-Affirming Way to Work and Become What You Really Desire by Jag Shoker

Have you lost your spark or the passion for what you do? Is your heart no longer in your work or (like so many people) are you simply disillusioned by the frantic race to get ahead in life? Your sense of unease may be getting harder to ignore, and comes from the growing urge to step off the treadmill and pursue a more thrilling and meaningful direction in life. *You Will Thrive* addresses the subject of modern disillusionment. It is essential reading for people looking to make the most of their talents and be something more in life. Something that matters. Something that makes a difference in the world. Through six empowering steps, it reveals 'the Way' to boldly follow your heart as it leads you to the perfect opportunities you seek.

The Winning Golf Swing: Simple Technical Solutions for Lower Scores by Kristian Baker

In *The Winning Golf Swing*, renowned golf professional Kristian Baker gives you a practical, yet easy-to-follow path to better golf. Through a rigorous but simple process, Kristian will help you to address the problems in your game so that you can shoot better scores. With contributions from some of the top minds in golf, this book delivers a complete process for improvement.

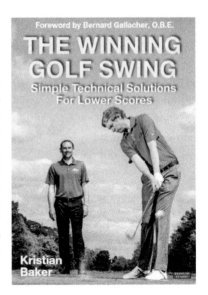

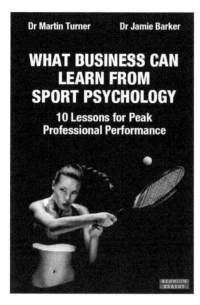

What Business Can Learn From Sport Psychology: Ten Lessons for Peak Professional Performance by Martin Turner and Jamie Barker

How are the best athletes in the world able to function under the immense pressure of competition? By harnessing the potential of their minds to train smart, stay committed, focus, and deliver winning performances with body and mind when the time is right.

In *What Business Can Learn From Sport Psychology* you will develop the most important weapon you need to succeed in business: your mental approach to performance. This book reveals the secrets of the winning mind by exploring the strategies and techniques used by the most successful athletes and professionals on the planet.

Aphantasia: Experiences, Perceptions, and Insights by Alan Kendle

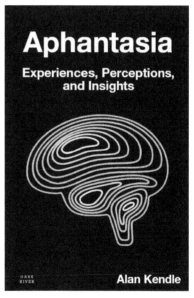

Close your eyes and picture a sunrise. For the majority of people, the ability to visualize images – such as a sunrise – seems straightforward, and can be accomplished 'on demand'. But, for potentially some 2% of the population, conjuring up an image in one's mind's eye is not possible; attempts to visualize images just bring up darkness.

Put together by lead author Alan Kendle – who discovered his Aphantasia in 2016 – this title is a collection of insights from contributors across the world detailing their lives with the condition. It offers rich, diverse, and often amusing insights and experiences into Aphantasia's effects. For anyone who wishes to understand this most intriguing condition better, the book provides a wonderful and succinct starting point.

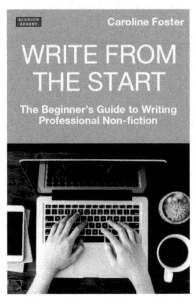

Write From The Start: The Beginner's Guide to Writing Professional Non-Fiction by Caroline Foster

Do you want to become a writer? Would you like to earn money from writing? Do you know where to begin?

Help is at hand with *Write From The Start* – a practical must-read resource for newcomers to the world of non-fiction writing. It is a vast genre that encompasses books, newspaper and magazine articles, press releases, business copy, the web, blogging, and much more besides. Jam-packed with great advice, the book is aimed at novice writers, hobbyist writers, or those considering a full-time writing career, and offers a comprehensive guide to help you plan, prepare, and professionally submit your non-fiction work. It is designed to get you up-and-running fast.

Finding Your Way Back to YOU: A self-help book for women who want to regain their Mojo and realise their dreams! by Lynne Saint

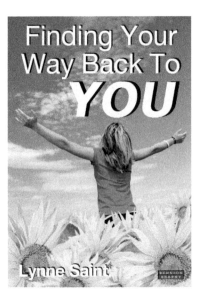

Are you at a crossroads in life, lacking in motivation, looking for a new direction or just plain 'stuck'? *Finding your Way back to YOU* is a focused and concise resource written specifically for women who have found themselves in any of the positions above.

Designed as a practical book with an accompanying downloadable journal and weblinked exercises, Finding Your Way Back to YOU is an inspiring book that introduces Neuro- Linguistic Programming, and Cognitive Behavioural Therapy techniques for change that are particularly valuable within the coaching context.

CPSIA information can be obtained
at www.ICGtesting.com
Printed in the USA
BVHW041054090419
545033BV00017B/679/P